Esophageal Cancer: Beyond Current Treatments

Sharlin

First Printing, 2024

Table of Contents

Chapter 1: General introduction

1.1 Esophageal squamous cell carcinoma

Esophageal cancer is a common malignancy which occurs in the esophagus, a muscular tract connecting the throat and the stomach. Mainly due to late diagnosis, esophageal cancer patients often present advanced staged tumors and thus a dismal overall 5-year survival rate of 19% (Siegel et al., 2019). Over the past decades, increased biological understanding of esophageal cancer and advances in health care have led to a better clinical outcome in different populations. More specifically, the overall 5-year survival rate has increased dramatically from less than 5% to around 20% during the last 50 years (Njei et al., 2016; Zeng et al., 2015). However, esophageal cancer still represents an aggressive disease entity comparing to prostate cancer, melanoma of the skin and female breast cancer whose overall 5-year survival rates are 98%, 92% and 90%, respectively (Siegel et al., 2019). Because of the limited treatment options for esophageal cancer, it remains a deadly malignancy, ranking as the sixth leading cause of cancer-related death worldwide (Fitzmaurice et al., 2015). This malignancy often leads to a significant decline in health-related quality of life (HRQoL) (Lagergren et al., 2017), thus highlighting the need for a better understanding of this cancer entity and the development of more effective therapies.

1.1.1 Epidemiology of esophageal squamous cell carcinoma

Histologically, there are two subtypes of esophageal cancer: esophageal squamous cell carcinoma (ESCC) and esophageal adenocarcinoma (EAC). Apart from distinct epidemiological and pathological characteristics, ESCC and EAC are associated with different risk factors which will be discussed in the following sections. The incidence trend of each subtype is also influenced by multiple factors, such as smoking, alcohol consumption and diet (Abnet et al., 2018; Smyth et al., 2017). Furthermore, ESCC and EAC have divergent molecular characteristics, where ESCC resembles head and neck squamous cell carcinoma (HNSCC) whereas EAC shares many genetic features with chromosomally unstable gastric adenocarcinoma (Kim et al., 2017). Therefore, ESCC and EAC have different epidemiological features and in this work ESCC will be our main focus.

1.1.1.1 Incidence

In 2012, about 398,000 individuals developed ESCC, and of these cases, 278,000 were men and 120,000 were women, indicating a higher risk for men (Arnold et al., 2015). Indeed, the male-to-female incidence ratio of ESCC is 2.7, which hints that differences between men and women play a role in the development of ESCC. Still, this gender dependency varies greatly among regions. For example, the male-to-female incidence ratio is significantly higher in low risk region (e.g. around 4:1 in USA) compared with high risk region (e.g. around 1:1 in China) (Arnold et al., 2015). Besides gender, the propensity to develop ESCC is also correlated with age, with the majority of ESCC and EAC patients being older people (Abnet et al., 2018). Fortunately, over the past few decades, the incidence of ESCC has declined substantially in many countries. For example, a continuous annual decrease (over 3%) of ESCC incidence was observed in both the USA and China from 1990s to mid-2000s (Trivers et al., 2008; Zhao et al., 2012) enabling EAC to become the predominant subtype in some regions and in many western countries, such as the UK and the USA. Nevertheless, ESCC remains the predominant histological subtype in many high risk regions including China which, by itself, has more than half of the ESCC cases (Arnold et al., 2015).

1.1.1.2 Geographical distribution of ESCC

It is very intriguing that different esophageal cancer subtypes predominate in distinct geographical locations – ESCC in Asia and Africa and EAC in Europe and America. There has been a long-standing esophageal cancer belt stretching from northern China through central Asia to northern Iran. This "belt" sees a particularly high incidence of ESCC (Fig. 1). More specifically, certain areas in central and northern China have an extremely high incidence rate, ranking among the highest incidence rates globally, where 100 in 100,000 people develop ESCC (Lin et al., 2013). In Linxian, a county in the Taihang mountains, 110 in 100,000 people develop ESCC, which also accounts for 20% of total deaths in the county. In the early 20th century, local residents in Linxian even built a temple named "Throat-God Temple" to pray that they would not develop esophageal cancer. This clearly reflects the impact of esophageal cancer in that particular area (Yang, 1980).

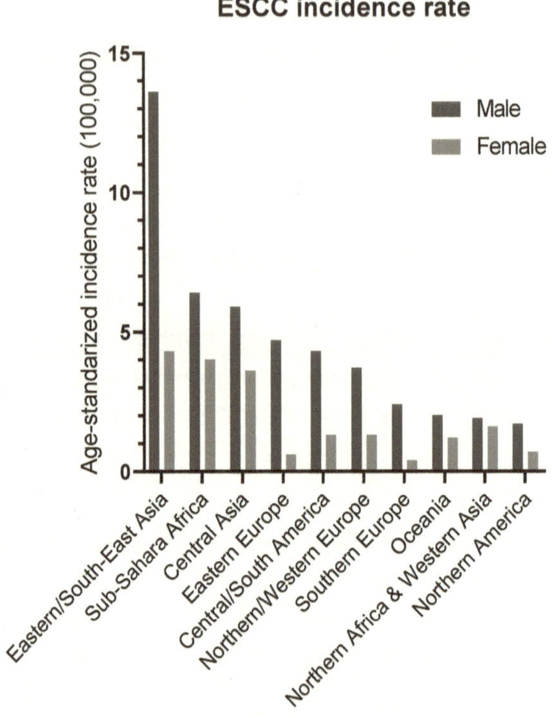

Fig. 1 ESCC incidence rates in different geographical locations. The incidence rate is exceptionally high in East Asia, but it is low in Europe and America. (Modified from (Arnold et al., 2015))

Moreover, the prevalence of ESCC is markedly lower in urban areas than in rural areas. For example, the age-standardized rate (ASR) of ESCC in Beijing, Shanghai and Guangzhou ranged from 9.2 to 10.2 in 100,000 people, being significantly lower than that in central rural areas in China such as Henan and Hebei (Lin et al., 2013). Although the incidence rate varies greatly within China, overall it is still much higher than in western countries and makes ESCC the fourth leading cause of cancer-related death in China. In western countries, EAC has surpassed ESCC to become the predominant subtype. Moreover, the incidence of EAC is still on the rise, while the incidence of ESCC has been declining over the past decades (Smyth et al., 2017). Collectively, these observations clearly show that ESCC has distinct incidence rates among different geographical areas and that people are more likely to develop ESCC in less industrialized regions, such as East Asia.

1.1.1.3 Risk factors

Risk factors are elements which increase the likelihood of developing a particular disease. Generally, aging, tobacco, alcohol, family history, viral or bacterial infection, radiation and certain chemicals are risk factors for cancer. In the scenario of ESCC, the etiology has also been studied extensively and many risk factors have been identified. Like the incidence of ESCC, risk factors contributing to ESCC development in different regions or populations also differ.

1.1.1.3.1 Tobacco

Tobacco smoke has several prominent carcinogens, such as polycyclic hydrocarbons, nitrosamines, aromatic amines. Active tobacco smoking has been correlated with high risk of ESCC development. More specifically, tobacco smokers have a five to nine times higher risk of developing ESCC compared to non-smokers (Freedman et al., 2007a). But the contribution of tobacco to the development of ESCC is largely limited to developed countries which are often low-incidence regions. On the contrary, tobacco smoking seemed to play a smaller role in high-incidence areas such as China. For example, in Linxian, which is among the high incidence regions, almost half of the ESCC patients were women but less than 1% of women smoked (Tran et al., 2005). However, tobacco smoking is still considered a risk factor even in high-incidence regions and the distinct relative risk of developing ESCC in current smokers in different regions remains to be addressed.

1.1.1.3.2 Alcohol

Alcohol has been reported to be a causative factor for the development of ESCC (Abnet et al., 2018). Acetaldehyde, the primary metabolite of ethanol metabolism, has been classified as a Class-I carcinogen and is widely acknowledged as a risk factor contributing to the development of ESCC (Ohashi et al., 2015). It can cause several different types of DNA (deoxyribonucleic acid) damage, which can potentially lead to carcinogenic mutations (Mizumoto et al., 2017; Seitz and Stickel, 2007). Apart from being a product of ethanol metabolism, acetaldehyde is also found in alcoholic beverages, increasing the exposure of the esophageal mucosa to acetaldehyde (Uebelacker and Lachenmeier, 2011). Similar to tobacco, the etiological contribution of alcohol to ESCC also varies in different regions with distinct incidence rates. In low-incidence areas, such as Europe and North America, the consumption of alcohol is tightly correlated with the incidence of ESCC (Garidou et al., 1996; Vaughan et al., 1995; Vioque et al., 2008). On the other hand, in high-incidence areas, such correlation is weaker. For example, in a cohort conducted in Linxian, no correlation was found between alcohol consumption and the incidence of ESCC (Tran et al., 2005). Notably, synergistic effects of tobacco and alcohol on the development of ESCC were observed in different cohorts (Prabhu et al., 2014; Sakata et al., 2005). In conclusion, alcohol consumption is a clear risk factor for ESCC except in regions with exceptionally high incidence rates.

1.1.1.3.3 Diet

Diet has also been suggested to play a role in the progression of ESCC. Due to the complexity of diet, many individual food or beverages have been examined with regard to ESCC and some of them correlated with an increased risk of malignancy in certain areas.

For example, the low intake of vegetables and fruits has been reported to increase the risk of developing ESCC (Freedman et al., 2007b; Yamaji et al., 2008). The anti-carcinogenesis role of vegetables and fruits can be partly attributed to the high concentration of micronutrients. This is further supported by a report conducted in a high-incidence region showing that the deprivation of minerals, such as selenium and zinc, as well as vitamins is associated with a higher risk of developing ESCC (Taylor et al., 1994). Different from alcohol or tobacco, the effects of vegetable and fruits on the development of ESCC are consistent despite different incidence rates in different regions (Levi et al., 2000; Riboli and Norat, 2003; Tran et al., 2005).

Pickled vegetables are an indispensable part of the diet of many Asian families. The process of vegetable pickling frequently generates nitrite and nitrate, which can further form carcinogenic compounds such as nitrosamines. Consistently, intake of pickled vegetables has been reported to increase the risk of developing ESCC (Liang et al., 2017). This is further supported by some animal experiments demonstrating the carcinogenic role of pickled vegetables (Lu et al., 1981).

Hot food and beverages have also been thought to be a causal factor for ESCC (Islami et al., 2009a). Consumption of hot food and beverages can potentially irritate the esophageal mucosa, thus weakening the defensive capacity of the esophageal epithelium. The temperature of hot food or beverages is critical for the development of ESCC as revealed by a study in which tea-drinking was not significantly associated with the risk of developing ESCC, whereas drinking tea at high temperature was positively associated with ESCC development in both ESCC high- and low-incidence regions in the Jiangsu province of China (Wu et al., 2009). Similarly, consumption of extremely hot beverages, i.e. > 70 °C, is correlated with a higher risk of developing ESCC in Iran (Islami et al., 2009b), Tanzania (Munishi et al., 2015), and Kenya (Middleton et al., 2019), high-incidence regions. Coffee, however, has not been shown to contribute to the carcinogenesis of ESCC and this could probably be explained by the fact that people rarely drink coffee at a temperature higher than 60 °C (Abnet et al., 2018).

1.1.1.3.4 Socioeconomic status

Socioeconomic status (SES) is a complex concept which covers many aspects of social and economic activities and conditions of individuals. More specifically, SES is a measure which takes education, occupation, income and several other factors into consideration. Interestingly, it is one of the most consistent risk factors for ESCC development in both high- and low-incidence regions. Developed or industrialized countries are almost all low ESCC incidence regions, which is in line with the fact that a better SES is inversely associated with the risk of developing ESCC. Such cases are seen in Sweden (Jansson et al., 2005) and the United States (Gammon et al., 1997). Consistently, in high-incidence regions, such as China, SES is also strongly associated with the risk of developing ESCC (Gao et al., 2018; Xibib et al., 2003). These findings shaped SES as a robust risk factor of ESCC which is more predictive than tobacco and alcohol. However, systematically determining SES and its consequences remains challenging.

1.1.1.3.5 Genetic variations

Genetic contribution to various diseases has been largely appreciated and significantly influences ESCC. Several genetic studies have shown evidence supporting the role of family history in the carcinogenesis of ESCC (Chen et al., 2015b; Gao et al., 2009).

The most prominent genetic variation associated with ESCC is a mutation in *RHDBF2*. This missense mutation can lead to tylosis, an autosomal dominant disorder with symptoms of palmar and plantar hyperkeratosis (Blaydon et al., 2012; Smyth et al., 2017). Most tylosis patients, up to 95%, develop ESCC before the age of 65, while the risk of developing other cancers is not altered in these patients (Ellis et al., 1994; Hennies et al., 1995; Stevens et al., 1996). The rapid development of next generation sequencing (NGS) has massively increased the throughput of biological assays. This technique also boosted the identification of genetic variations (e.g. single nucleotide polymorphism (SNP)) associated with many diseases achieved by genome-wide association studies (GWAS) which directly led to a better stratification of disease-associated risk (Tam et al., 2019). Utilizing GWAS, several genetic loci associated with risk of ESCC development in Chinese populations were identified and are summarized in Table 1 (Abnet et al., 2012; Wang et al., 2010; Wu et al., 2011, 2012a, 2014). The nearest genes were listed, but it is worth noting that they are not necessarily associated with those SNPs, as, for example, variations within regulatory elements can regulate distal genes.

Table 1 SNPs associated with increased risk of ESCC development among Chinese

SNP	Locus	Associated genes	OR	Reference
rs2274223	10q23	*PLCE1*	1.43	Wang *et al.*, 2010
rs11066015	12q24	*ALDH2*	1.38	Wu *et al.*, 2011
rs10484761	6p21	*UNC5CL*	1.33	Wu *et al.*, 2011
rs11066280	12q24	*RPL6, PTPN11*	1.3	Wu *et al.*, 2011
rs2074356	12q24	*C12orf51*	1.56	Wu *et al.*, 2011
rs1042026	4q23	*ADH1B*	1.35	Wu *et al.*, 2012
rs13016963	10q23	*CASP8, ALS2CR12*	1.29	Abnet *et al.*, 2012
rs35597309	6p21	HLA Class II genes	1.19	Wu *et al.*, 2014

OR: odds ratio.

PLCE1 (Phospholipase C Epsilon 1) encodes a phospholipase which contains binding domains for Ras proteins and acts downstream of GTPase-mediated signaling pathways. Through binding to small Ras GTPases, PLCE1 relays oncogenic signaling during the progression of HNSCC (Bunney et al., 2009), a cancer entity resembling the molecular characteristics of ESCC. In addition, PLCE1 has also been shown to promote the carcinogenesis of skin and intestinal malignancies (Bai et al., 2004; Li et al., 2009b), highlighted the oncogenic function of this protein as well as the necessity for further research on PLCE1.

Alcohol has been identified as a risk factor for the development of ESCC, as previously mentioned (in section 1.1.1.3.2). The synergistic effects between functional variants of *ALDH2* (Aldehyde Dehydrogenase 2) and *ADH1B* (Alcohol Dehydrogenase 1B), two alcohol metabolizing enzymes, and tobacco smoking in promoting the development of ESCC has also been reported (Cui et al., 2009). The variants associated with *ALDH2* and *ADH1B* were also over-represented in ESCC cases in large scale GWAS studies (Wu et al., 2011, 2012a). Another study showed that people carrying these variants and overconsuming alcohol had a 73-fold higher risk of developing ESCC, while subjects carrying the same variants and drinking moderate amounts of alcohol had a lower risk of developing ESCC (Yokoyama et al., 2003).

Another interesting finding is that SNPs associated with HLA (Human Leukocyte Antigen) class II genes were found to be linked to higher risk of ESCC development in the Taihang mountains, a region in China with a high ESCC incidence rate (Wu et al., 2014). However, this association was only identified in the high-incidence region in China, which made the conclusion implausible. Genomic regions in close proximity to HLA class II genes, to rs35597309, have been associated with multiple cancers including lung cancer (Lan et al., 2012) and liver cancer (Li et al., 2012), which makes this genomic region of great interest for future research on the etiology of ESCC.

Recently, some SNPs have been tested in different regions with high ESCC incidence rates and a high degree of heterogeneity among the tested individuals was found (Bye et al., 2012). This finding suggests that SNPs identified from a certain region or race could be specific and potentially not applicable to other regions or races. Further examination of people in high-incidence regions will likely reveal valuable region-specific susceptibility genomic loci (e.g. rs35597309 in Taihang mountains). Moreover, genetic variations often pose vulnerabilities to specific environmental cues, thus enhancing the carcinogenesis of ESCC. One such example are variations associated with *ALDH2* and *ADH1B*, which synergized with smoking to enhance the risk of ESCC development (Cui et al., 2009). Therefore, such multifactorial design of experiments should be applied to further understand the etiology of ESCC.

1.1.2 Pathogenesis of ESCC

ESCC often occurs in the upper part of the esophagus (Fig. 2A), while EAC is usually diagnosed in the lower part, sometimes even in close proximity to the stomach. According to a study, in an ESCC cohort consisting of 1317 patients, 75.5% of patients were diagnosed with ESCC located in the upper 2/3 part of the esophagus (Jiang et al., 2015).

ESCC often originates in the esophageal epithelium and upon recurrent exposure to some risk factors, such as tobacco, alcohol and thermal irritation, hyperplasia can occur in the upper layer of epithelium. Over prolonged exposure to risk factors, squamous hyperplasia can progress to squamous dysplasia and finally to highly invasive ESCC. At a later stage, ESCC can invade through the submucosa and reach the adventitia. The underlying genetic changes are not fully understood yet, but some prominent mutations have been identified during the progression from hyperplasia, via dysplasia, to ESCC. By comparing dysplasia (intraepithelial neoplasia (IEN)) with ESCC samples, some genes harboring shared mutations were identified. Among them, were genes associated with DNA repair, apoptosis, proliferation and cell adhesion. Amongst the dysregulated genes, *TP53* (Tumor Protein p53), *CDKN2A* (Cyclin Dependent Kinase Inhibitor 2A) and *RB1* (Retinoblastoma Transcriptional Corepressor 1) were found to be associated with loss of heterozygosity (LOH) which leads to loss of function for the affected allele. Several genes, such as *CCND1* (Cyclin D1), *SOX2* (SRY-box transcription factor 2) and *MYC* (MYC proto-oncogene), were associated with copy number alterations (CNA) and their expression was elevated in both precancerous dysplasia and ESCC. With the knowledge about the mutation landscape, a seemingly plausible model is that the combination of the loss of *TP53*, *CDKN2A* and *RB1* and the gain of *CCND1*, *SOX2* and *MYC* leads to accumulated mutations, DNA damage and genomic instability, which contribute to carcinogenesis (Liu et al., 2017).

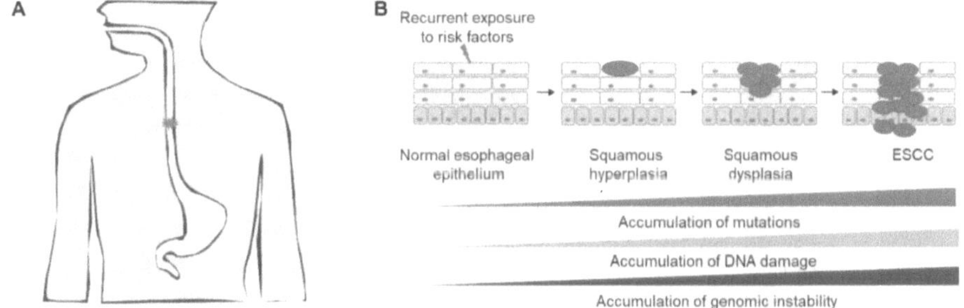

Fig. 2 Pathogenesis of ESCC. A: Scheme showing the location of ESCC. ESCC often occurs in the middle to upper esophageal tract, but it can also occur in the lower part and the gastroesophageal junction. B: The pathogenesis of ESCC. The recurrent exposure of esophagus to risk factors leads to squamous hyperplasia. Without medical intervention, squamous hyperplasia can develop to squamous dysplasia and ultimately to ESCC. At the molecular level, DNA damage, mutations and genomic instability together contribute to the development of ESCC.

1.1.3 Molecular characteristics of ESCC

Characterizing a disease at the molecular level is not only crucial for understanding the disease entity but also important for developing clinical approaches for prevention and intervention. The prognosis for ESCC remains dismal, highlighting the need for the development of novel therapies. Holding the principle that a better biological understanding could lead to a more effective therapy, several groups have utilized the NGS technique to investigate the molecular characteristics of ESCC (Gao et al., 2014; Kim et al., 2017; Lin et al., 2014; Sawada et al., 2016; Song et al., 2014). Consequently, the genomic, transcriptiomic and epigenomic landscapes of ESCC have been profiled which has led to a better biological understanding of ESCC. Prominent dysregulated genes are summarized in Fig. 3. These results suggest that ESCC has a distinct molecular profiling from EAC and shares many molecular features with squamous cell carcinoma originating from other anatomic sites such as HNSCC (Gao et al., 2014; Song et al., 2014).

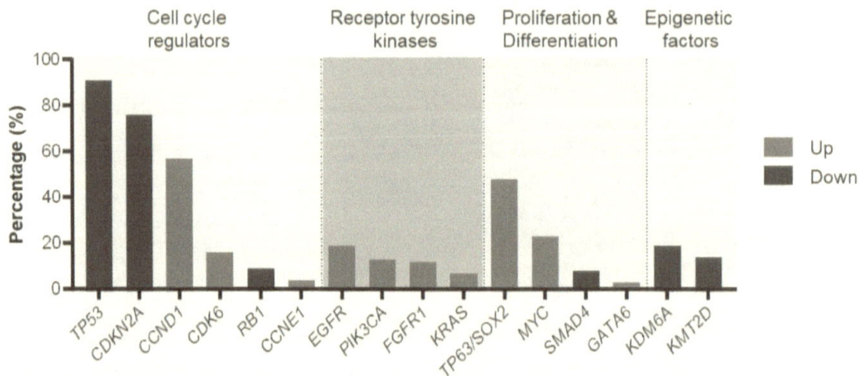

Fig. 3 Dysregulated genes in a cohort of ESCC (Kim et al., 2017). Genes up-regulated (Up) shown in red and genes down-regulated (Down) shown in blue. Negative regulators of cell cycle are often mutated such as *TP53* and *CDKN2A*, whereas positive regulators are likely to be amplified such as *CCND1*. Receptor tyrosine receptor pathways are also hyperactive. Transcription factors that are important for squamous-lineage-specification, such as *TP63* and *SOX2*, are largely amplified. The amplification of the MYC oncogene can provide cells with growth advantage. Moreover, some epigenetic factors are also mutated in a significant portion of ESCC.

1.1.3.1 Cell cycle regulators

Among dysregulated genes, *TP53* and *CDKN2A* have the highest mutation rates and their genetic alterations often lead to loss of function. The role of p53, "the guardian of the genome", in cancer has been intensively studied and p53 has been regarded as one of the most, if not the most, important tumor suppressor (Levine and Oren, 2009). p53 has been reported to function in DNA repair, cell cycle arrest and apoptosis, processes whose dysregulation is important for cancer progression (Riley et al., 2008). In the context of cell cycle regulation, p53 activates p21, a cyclin-dependent kinase inhibitor which interacts with the complex of cyclin-dependent kinase 4 (CDK4) and CycD1, leading to G1/S arrest (el-Deiry et al., 1993; Harper et al., 1993). p16, encoded by *CDKN2A*, can inhibit CDK4/CDK6-Cyclin D axis to subsequently promote the binding of RB1 to E2F, which ultimately leads to G1/S arrest (Hamilton and Infante, 2016; Sherr and Roberts, 2004). Interestingly, genomic regions associated with cyclins (*CCND1* and *CCNE1*) and cyclin-dependent kinases (*CDK6* (Cyclin-Dependent Kinase 6)) are often amplified, leading to elevated expression of these genes (Kim et al., 2017). ESCC cells can then utilize either or both of these genetic events to push cells through the G1/S checkpoint to gain a proliferative advantage over normal cells. In addition, mutations of p53 can convert it into an oncoprotein with increased stability and rewired transactivation activities, which can potentially enhance oncogenic properties (Mantovani et al., 2019).

1.1.3.2 Receptor tyrosine kinases

Receptor tyrosine kinases (RTKs) were discovered three decades ago and many of them have been shown to regulate key cellular processes such as cell proliferation, differentiation and migration (Ullrich and Schlessinger, 1990). RTKs are highly conserved and often consist of one extracellular domain responsible for ligand binding, one transmembrane domain and one intracellular domain including a tyrosine kinase domain. Depending on the ligand, RTKs were classified into different subfamilies including epidermal growth factor receptors (EGFRs), vascular endothelial growth factor receptors (VEGFRs) and fibroblast growth factor receptors (FGFRs) (Hubbard and Miller, 2007) (Fig. 4). In ESCC, various genes involved in EGFR and FGFR signaling pathways were affected (Fig. 3). In an ESCC cohort, 78% of patients had genetic alterations in genes which are downstream of EGFR signaling pathway, such as *KRAS*, *AKT1* and *PIK3CA* (Song et al., 2014). The hyperactive EGFR signaling pathway could account, at least in part, for the invasiveness of ESCC, thus also representing a therapeutic target. Indeed, there are already several RTK inhibitors, such as trastuzumab (Bang et al., 2010) and ramucirumab (Fuchs et al., 2018), approved by the FDA (Food and Drug Administration) for clinical use in gastroesophageal cancers.

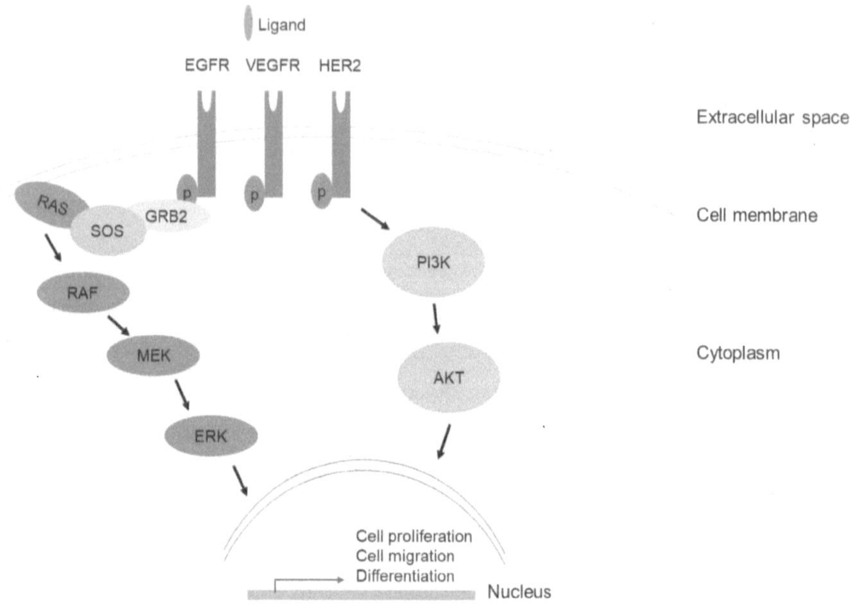

Fig. 4 A simplified scheme of RTK signaling pathway. Upon the binding of ligand, the receptor tyrosine kinases, such as EGFR, undergo autophosphorylation. The activation will then be passed on to MEK-ERK pathway (shown in purple) or PI3K-AKT pathway (shown in orange) to ultimately regulate gene expression.

1.1.3.3 Proliferation- and differentiation-related transcription factors

Cancer cells often undergo cellular transformation involving transcription factors (TF), which is also reflected by the transcriptional addiction of cancer cells (Bradner et al., 2017). MYC is a transcription factor with super strong transcriptional activities which are estimated to cover 15% of the entire human genome (Dang et al., 2006). Therefore, MYC is involved in a wide spectrum of cellular processes including cell proliferation, cell cycle regulation and cell migration (Chen et al., 2018). In ESCC, the *MYC* locus is amplified in more than 20% of cases (Fig. 3).

Another gene which is frequently dysregulated in ESCC is *SOX2*, a transcription factor described to be crucial for development and whose depletion is lethal (Avilion et al., 2003). It is most well known as a Yamanaka factor, because it can reprogram cells to generate induced pluripotent stem cells (iPSCs) in combination with three other transcription factors (Takahashi and Yamanaka, 2006). Furthermore, *SOX2* has been reported to be amplified in squamous cell carcinoma (SCC) drawing a lot of interest and leading to several functional studies of SOX2 in cancer biology (Bass et al., 2009). For example, SOX2 has been reported to interact with p63 inducing a specific transcription program and consequently maintaining the squamous cell lineage in SCC models (Watanabe et al., 2014). For this reason, SOX2 is regarded as an oncoprotein in ESCC.

Similar to *SOX2*, the *TP63* locus is frequently amplified in SCC, implicating its oncogenic role in SCC (Rocco et al., 2006; Sawada et al., 2016). *TP63* encodes two primary categories of isoforms – TAp63 and ΔNp63 and each of them has several different isoforms (Murray-Zmijewski et al., 2006). TAp63, the protein output of the full length *TP63*, contains a transactivation domain and is mainly expressed in oocytes (Suh et al., 2006), while the expression of ΔNp63, lacking the N-terminal transactivation domain, is normally restricted to the epidermis (Mills et al., 1999) (Fig. 5).

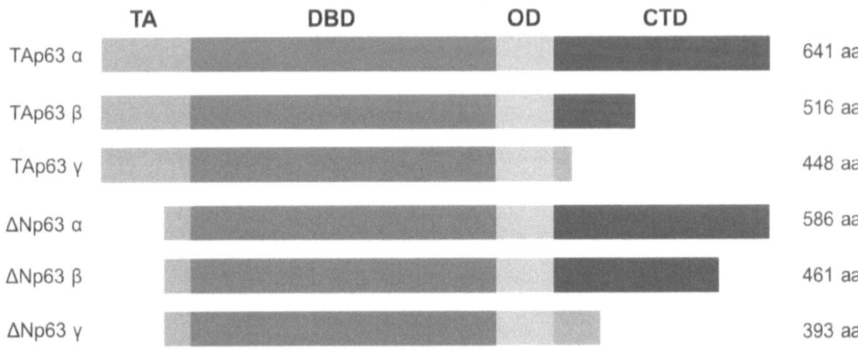

Fig. 5 Isoform structure of p63. TA: Transactivation domain; DBD: DNA-binding domain; OD: oligomerization domain; CTD: C-terminus domain. Modified from (Murray-Zmijewski et al., 2006).

Interestingly, both isoforms were classified as members of the p53 family because of their high homology (Yang et al.). In fact, TAp63 functions in cell cycle regulation and apoptosis (Gressner et al., 2005), inducing cell cycle arrest upon DNA damage, resembling the function of p53 (Yang and McKeon, 2000). Furthermore, studies have shown that the loss of TAp63 leads to an increased metastatic potential in bladder cancer (Koga et al., 2003). Therefore, similarly to p53, TAp63 is widely accepted as a tumor suppressor. On the other hand, ΔNp63 is described to have an oncogenic role, as it can activate the expression of extracellular matrix (ECM) components to influence the tumor microenvironment, which can have substantial effects on tumor metastasis (Gatti et al., 2019). Furthermore, ΔNp63 can also regulate cell adhesion genes and consequently potentially influence cell migration (Yang et al., 2006). This suggests that these two isoforms, albeit being translated from the same genomic locus, have distinct biological functions.

Although lacking a large portion of the transactivation domain, ΔNp63 can still transcriptionally activate its target genes. The integrity of the DNA-binding domain of ΔNp63 enables its DNA-binding activity. Due to the high homology with p53, ΔNp63 can compete with p53 for binding at p53 target loci in the context of cancer in which p53 is frequently mutated. This way, ΔNp63 can abolish the function of the rarely remaining wild-type p53 to exert its oncogenic roles (Yang and McKeon, 2000). Moreover, ΔNp63 has been reported to directly bind and transcriptionally activate nearly 1,000 genes. More strikingly, 20% of these targets are transcription factors which can then activate more downstream targets, thus forming a transcriptional network dependent on ΔNp63 (Yang et al., 2006). Recently, a study from our group in pancreatic ductal adenocarcinoma (PDAC) reinforced this idea, as ΔNp63 was found to bind squamous-subtype-specific super enhancers (SEs) to control genes, which are essential for maintaining the squamous phenotype. Those genes also comprise subtype-specific transcription factors (TFs) such as BHLHE40, RXRA and HIF1A, which can subsequently regulate downstream genes, forming an interconnected network contributing to cell phenotype (Hamdan and Johnsen, 2018). ΔNp63 is overexpressed in many cancers, especially in SCCs, hinting at its role in driving the squamous subtype in several cancer entities (Melino, 2011; Sniezek et al., 2004). Taken together, these findings suggest that ΔNp63 utilizes its wide spectrum of target genes and inhibitory effects of wild-type p53 to sustain tumor cell survival, while promoting the transcription of lineage-specific TFs driving the squamous subtype in different cancers. It further highlights how the dysregulation of different transcription factors in SCC and ESCC can promote tumorigenesis and affect tumor phenotype.

1.1.3.4 Epigenetic factors

The dysregulation of epigenetic factors has been recognized as a hallmark of cancer progression, displaying a high potential for clinical intervention (Morel et al., 2020). In

ESCC, several epigenetic factors including *KDM6A* (Lysine Demethylase 6A), *KMT2D* (Lysine Methyltransferase 2D) and *EP300* (E1A Binding Protein P300, a histone acetyltransferase) are mutated, indicating their tumor suppressor function (Gao et al., 2014; Song et al., 2014). In fact, *KDM6A* is mutated in many cancer types including bladder cancer (Nickerson et al., 2014), kidney cancer (Dalgliesh et al., 2010), leukemia (Jankowska et al., 2011) and prostate cancer (Grasso et al., 2012). In ESCC, UTX, the protein product of *KDM6A*, has been shown to regulate epithelial to mesenchymal transition (EMT). The loss of UTX led to increased cell proliferation and EMT, measured by increased levels of Vimentin and decreased levels of E-cadherin (Li et al., 2018). Similarly, *KMT2D* is also frequently mutated in various cancers (Rao and Dou, 2015) and its tumor suppressive function has been reported in lung cancer (Alam et al., 2020) and prostate cancer (Lv et al., 2018). Conversely, *EP300* is mutated in more than 10% of ESCC, but it has been reported to promote cell proliferation, colony formation, migration and invasion, suggesting the mutations could activate the p300-related program. Moreover, the expression of p300 is also correlated with poor prognosis, supporting an oncogenic role in ESCC (Bi et al., 2019). The high mutation rate and the oncogenic function highlighted the importance of p300 in ESCC, thus necessitating studies of specific mutations p300 and their biological consequences.

Collectively, these molecular characteristics revealed by genome-wide studies have greatly advanced our knowledge on ESCC and led to many clinical implications.

1.1.4 Treatment options

The choice of treatment for ESCC is primarily dependent on the stage. The general principle is that endoscopic treatment is recommended for earlier stages, surgery with or without chemotherapy is recommended for middle stages and curative or palliative chemotherapy is recommended for late stages (Lagergren et al., 2017). Precision medicine approaches have also been explored and may have a great potential for improving the prognosis of ESCC.

1.1.4.1 Endoscopic treatment

Patients who are diagnosed at early stages of EAC with minimal invasion to surrounding tissue are likely to benefit from endoscopic treatment. This has been applied to early EAC patients, but it has a good potential for treating ESCC patients as well. What is disappointing is that this category of patients (early stage with no or minimal invasion to the basal layer of esophageal mucosa) only makes up a small portion. With the advances in endoscopy and the intensified healthcare and medical surveillance, more patients with early stages of esophageal cancer can be diagnosed and receive endoscopic treatment (Smyth et al., 2017).

1.1.4.2 Chemotherapy and surgery

Surgical resection remains the recommended treatment option for more advanced patients. Although endoscopic treatment can be applied in certain cases and often results in better HRQoL, surgical treatment has been proven to have a lower recurrence rate (Lagergren et al., 2017). Locally advanced patients are often recommended for surgery following chemotherapy or chemoradiotherapy to optimize prognosis. A randomized control trial has compared the effects of surgery followed by chemotherapy treatment or not and concluded that cisplatin and fluorouracil followed by surgery significantly improved survival (Allum et al., 2009). However, there are also studies showing that patients treated with only chemotherapy have similar survival rates when compared to patients undergoing surgery and adjuvant chemotherapy, suggesting that surgery may not be needed in certain cases (Bedenne et al., 2007; Stahl et al., 2005). Thus, proper staging of ESCC patients is essential for the decision on treatment.

1.1.4.3 Precision medicine

Precision medicine is a term used to describe tailored medical practices which take into account the differences among patients including genetic background, family history as well as psychosocial and phenotypic characteristics (Fig. 6) (Jameson and Longo, 2015). In fact, the uniqueness of individuals is not only the core requirement, but also the power of precision medicine. Precision medicine is not a new term, and people actually started practicing it before conceptualizing this term. For example, when a blood transfusion is needed, the clinician will do a test to see if the blood type of the donor and the recipient match In this case, the physiological characteristic, i.e. blood type, of the donor and recipient has been considered and this has guided the clinician to make the right decision. The concept of subgrouping individuals has been well appreciated in this scenario. However, we should not ignore the fact that this is all based on our scientific knowledge on blood types. Therefore, understanding a disease from all possible aspects is not only beneficial for basic science research, but also for clinical approaches.

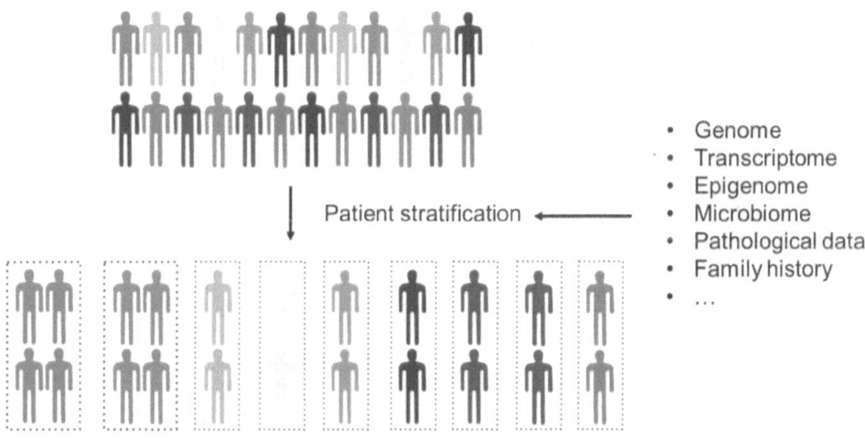

Fig. 6 Scheme showing the principle of precision medicine. Patients with different characteristics are shown in different colors. Multiple factors (shown in the light blue rectangle) are used to stratify patients and different subgroups of patients get tailored therapies according to their specific background.

Since the sequencing of the human genome (Venter et al., 2001), the uniqueness of human beings has been well appreciated simply because it is highly unlikely for two individuals to share exactly the same three billion base pairs of DNA. By understanding the human genome and its biological function better, we can now use some of the findings as criteria to refine our stratification system to guide the medical doctors toward an evidence-based treatment for patients (Ginsburg and Phillips, 2018). The rapid development of sequencing technologies has greatly increased sequencing capacity and decreased cost. Today, there are many "sequencing factories" around the globe which are operating at low costs. Many hospitals and research institutes even have their own sequencing facilities, which facilitates the development of precision medicine. Given all the advances that have been made in the field of precision medicine, a general framework of precision medicine has shaped up (Fig. 7). In this system, patients and clinicians report the clinical data to the information database, which is patient-specific. The biological samples collected from patients is transferred to researchers who then conduct various investigations including 2D/3D cell culture, animal model establishment, genome, transcriptome, epigenome sequencing and drug sensitivity screening. These results are then integrated with the clinical data to further characterize the patient. With help from a vast curated knowledge base, a personalized medical decision based on the patient's profile is then provided to the patient. The response of the patient to the given treatment is documented and integrated into the database, which can in turn strengthen the knowledge database.

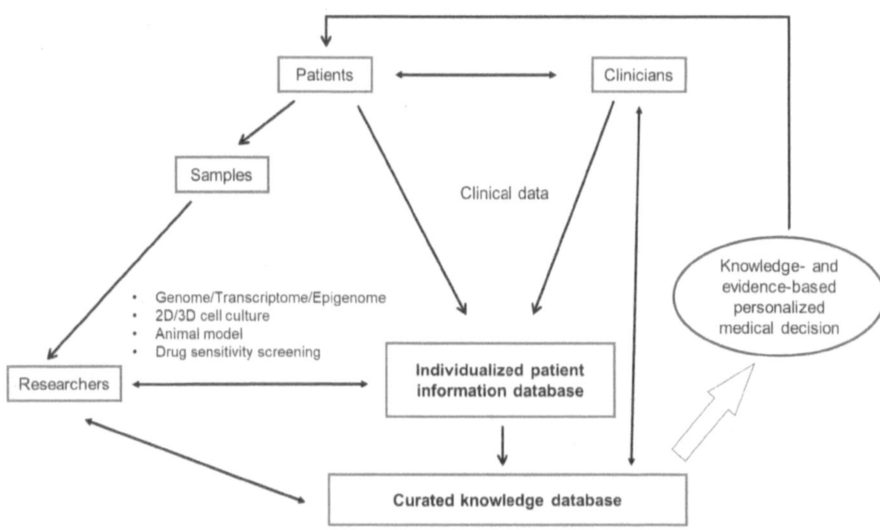

Fig. 7 A proposed workflow of precision medicine. Modified from (Aronson and Rehm, 2015). Upon enrolling, patients and clinicians collect the clinical data and store it in a database. Biopsies are collected and used for sequencing, drug sensitivity screening, etc. Combing the lab result, clinical data and the curated knowledge, a tailored treatment is then recommended for patients.

There are already some successful examples showing that targeting the underlying molecular alterations can have a better clinical outcome (Kumar-Sinha and Chinnaiyan, 2018). One famous example is the application of Imatinib, an agent inhibiting the causative Bcr-Abl oncopeotein, in chronic myeloid leukemia (CML), which highlighted the potential of targeted therapy (Mauro et al., 2001). However, the complexity of the cancer genome is extensive. The high degree of heterogeneity and complex genome of tumors slowed the development of precision medicine (Prasad et al., 2016), suggesting continuous efforts should be made to decode the complex genome of each molecularly-distinct cancer subtype in order to identify novel therapeutic targets.

In ESCC, there have been some advances in developing targeted therapies. Main molecular targets of the RTK signaling pathway have been tested including, but not limited to, EGFR and HER2 (Belkhiri and El-Rifai, 2015). In fact, many of the recent clinical trials of targeted therapies in ESCC (with the exception of immunotherapy which will be discussed later) focus on EGFR, probably due to the recurrent dysregulation of EGFR signaling in ESCC (Gao et al., 2014; Kim et al., 2017; Lin et al., 2014; Sawada et al., 2016; Song et al., 2014). Despite several clinical trials involving different EGFR inhibitors, such as Nimotuzumab (NCT02011594, NCT01993784 and NCT01232374), Icotinib (NCT01973725) and Gefitinib (NCT01291823, NCT00258323) in ESCC, no study has proven successful Furthermore, targeted therapies against FGFR (Van Cutsem et al., 2017), VEGFR (Ohtsu et al., 2011), mTOR (Mechanistic Target of Rapamycin) (Ohtsu et al., 2013) and HGFR (Hepatocyte Growth Factor Receptor) (Shah et al., 2017) were also tested for the treatment of esophageal cancer. A limitation of such studies was that most of these patients were diagnosed with EAC, such that no decisive conclusion can be drawn regarding the usage of such inhibitors in the treatment of ESCC.

Still, HER2 inhibition has shown promising results in several studies, being regarded as a potential target in the treatment of ESCC. In a preclinical study, a patient derived xenograft (PDX) model was used to test the anti-tumor effects of Trastuzumab, a monoclonal antibody that targets the extracellular domain of HER2. In this case, HER2-positive PDX models showed a tumor regression upon receiving Tratuzumab treatment (Wu et al., 2012b). Moreover, a randomized controlled trial has also shown that using Tratuzumab along with chemotherapy can increase the median overall survival (OS) in gastro-esophageal junction cancer (Bang et al., 2010). Thus, Tratuzumab may be a potential candidate for the treatment of ESCC patients. Future clinical studies with more ESCC patients are needed to determine the efficacy of this promising drug in ESCC.

Besides targeting RTK pathways, immunotherapy has also been tested in ESCC. In one study, ESCC patients who were positive for PDL1 (Programmed Cell Death

Protein 1 Ligand 1) received pembrolizumab, an antibody which binds to and blocks PD1 (Programmed Cell Death Protein 1) located on the surface of T-cell. These patients displayed an impressive objective response rate of 29% (Doi et al., 2016). In another clinical study, of a PDL1-unselected ESCC cohort (64 patients), 17% of the patients showed a response to the anti-PD1 monoclonal antibody nivolumab (Kudo et al., 2017). These promising results have led to more clinical tests of immunotherapeutic agents in ESCC and there are currently 14 such clinical trials

~~There are also some other~~ targets which can be of clinical value, such as the frequently dysregulated CDK6. Clinical trials testing CDK4/CDK6 inhibition in ESCC are also ongoing (NCT04000529 and NCT03292250).

Overall, there are some advances in developing targeted therapies for ESCC, but, unfortunately, no satisfactory results were obtained yet. Moreover, the lack of validated therapeutic targets has slowed down the process of developing anti-tumor drugs. Therefore, it is of critical importance to identify new potential therapeutic targets for the development of targeted therapies in ESCC.

1.2. Epigenetic regulation and dysregulation

1.2.1 Epigenetics

The coordination of activities in human beings is highly complex, considering the high degree and interconnectivity of communication and coordination needed among organs and tissues. Even at the cellular level, biological events, such as replication, transcription and translation are very well controlled under a complicated and systematic regulatory mechanism. Genetic material that is passed on over generations is an essential factor contributing to the homeostasis of cells. Genetic material is highly stable and universal across the human body with the exception of germline cells. However, the environment we live in is not constantly stable, requiring cells to act rapidly to adapt to environmental stimuli. Epigenetics is one such mechanism that cells use to integrate environmental stimuli and the intrinsic regulation network to maintain homeostasis. Introduced by Conrad Waddington in the 1940s, epigenetics was defined as "the branch of biology which studies the causal interactions between genes and their products which bring the phenotype into being" (Waddington, 1942), as described in Fig. 8. The concept of epigenetics has been modified over the last decades and now it mainly refers to a subject which studies changes in gene expression which do not entail a change in DNA sequence (Wu and Morris, 2001). Epigenetic changes can happen at different levels of genome organization, such as DNA, histone and chromatin spatial organization. The detail of each epigenetic change will be discussed in the following sections. Epigenetic changes are often reversible due to the existence of three groups of epigenetic factors: epigenetic writers (responsible for catalyzing epigenetic modifications), erasers (responsible for removing epigenetic modifications) and readers (responsible for interpreting epigenetic modifications). Depending on the type of modification, epigenetic factors for "writing", "erasing" and "interpreting" also differ.

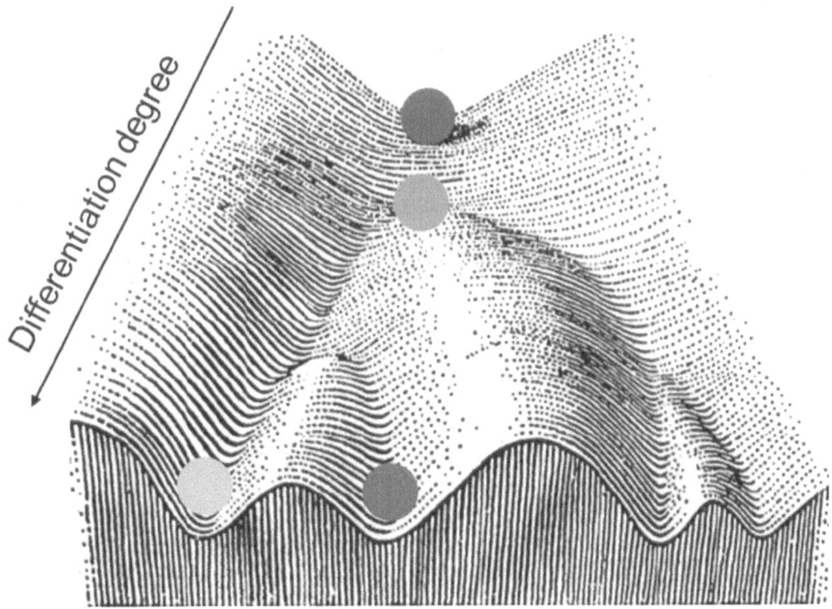

Fig. 8 Scheme of Waddington Model. Cells with pluripotency become differentiated cells and lose stem cell properties during the differentiation process. Modified from (Baedke, 2013).

1.2.2 Genome organization

The human genome, roughly estimated to be around 2 meters (m) in length, is packaged in a nucleus with an average diameter at the micrometer (μm) scale. This means that the genome has to be condensed and folded to a great extent and in a right order, which requires a multi-level regulatory mechanism. DNA, a double helix structure, is wrapped 1.7 turns around a histone octamer which consists of two each of H2A (Histone H2A), H2B (Histone H2B), H3 (Histone H3) and (Histone H4), forming a basic unit of chromatin - the nucleosome. Two nucleosomes, in turn, are connected by a complex of DNA and linker histone H1 (H1) (Zhou et al., 1998). The process of DNA wrapping around nucleosomes can provide a five to ten-time compaction of DNA (Kornberg, 1974). Furthermore, the DNA wrapped around the nucleosome provides substantially different accessibility to various DNA segments, such that TFs interact with distinct DNA regions which can potentially lead to changes in gene expression. Moreover, the "tail" of histones, nucleosome extruding peptides, can also be post-translationally modified by epigenetic "writers" to exert distinct regulatory functions. Furthermore, neighboring nucleosomes are further folded into a condensed chromatin fiber with a diameter of around 30 nanometer (nm) (Robinson et al., 2006). This condensed structure can often be folded again forming topologically associated domains (TADs) in which DNA-DNA contact is frequent. These different TADs can then be arranged to form two types of compartments: compartment A and compartment B. Compartment A is transcriptionally active while compartment B is transcriptionally inactive (Lieberman-Aiden et al., 2009; Wang et al., 2016). Finally, these compartments will then be packed in the nucleus in an ordered manner. Taken together, the multi-level hierarchy of the human genome is not the key for chromatin compaction but also the basis for gene regulation.

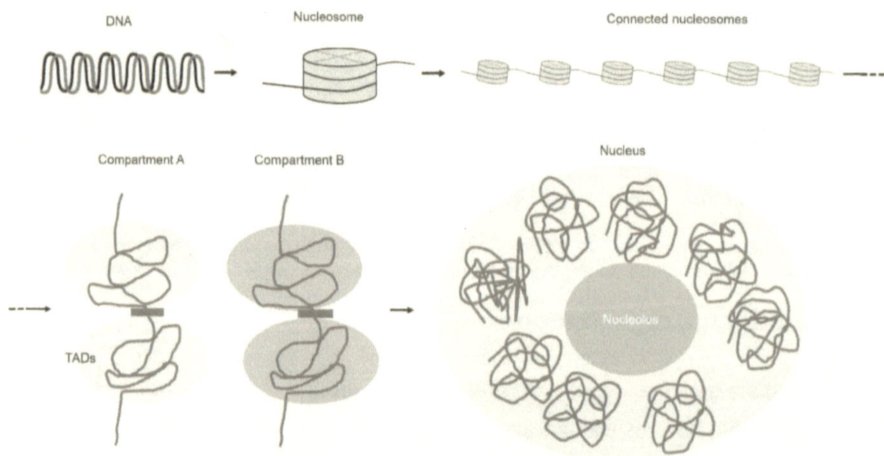

Fig. 9 Simplified scheme showing the hierarchical organization of genome. DNA is wrapped around the core histone octamer, forming a nucleosome. Nucleosomes are connected and folded forming topologically associated domains (TADs) in which frequent chromatin interaction occurs. TADs are further compacted into different compartments with distinct transcriptional activities. Compartments are packed and distributed in the nucleus.

1.2.3 The epigenetic code

The hierarchical organization of the human genome not only ensures the proper and maximal compaction, but also allows for regulation at different levels, which greatly diversifies gene regulation mechanisms and gene expression patterns. DNA modifications together with post-translational histone modifications compose the epigenetic code and shape gene regulation by affecting DNA accessibility and therefore the binding and recruitment of gene regulatory elements.

1.2.3.1 DNA methylation

DNA methylation is prevalently found in CpG (cytosine-guanine) dinucleotides and considered a repressive mark of gene expression (Holliday and Pugh, 1975; Riggs, 1975). In this case, methylation is mostly present on cytosine, more specifically on its 5th carbon yielding 5-methylcytosine (5mC). DNA methylation has been shown to play a critical role in development (Okano et al., 1999), while global DNA hypomethylation is one of the hallmarks of cancer (Baylin and Jones, 2016), suggesting its role in cancer progression. Furthermore, DNA methylation requires three groups of factors for three different processes: *de novo* DNA methylation, maintenance and demethylation. DNMT3A (DNA Methyltransferase 3A) and DNMT3B (DNA Methyltransferase 3B) are two major enzymes establishing methylation (Okano et al., 1998, 1999) and DNMT1 (DNA Methyltransferase 1) is required for the maintenance of DNA methylation upon DNA replication (Takeshita et al., 2011). DNA demethylation is a complex process involving consecutive oxidization steps of 5mC followed by DNA repair mechanisms. Methylcytosine dioxygenases, such as TETs (Ten-Elven Translocation), oxidize 5mC and the oxidized intermediates of 5mC are excised via DNA base excision repair ultimately achieving DNA demethylation (Bhutani et al., 2010).

Because DNA hypomethylation is a common feature in cancer, targeting the DNA methylation process was initially not considered to be a good strategy. However, many follow-up studies showed that many tumor suppressors gain methylation on their TSS during carcinogenesis (Issa, 2007; Toyota and Issa, 2005). Furthermore, mouse models have shown that a drop in DNA methylation decreased tumor formation (Belinsky et al., 2003; Laird et al., 1995). In conclusion, even though it is counterintuitive at first glance, patients may benefit from targeting DNA methylation. Still, there are currently very few clinical trials intended to test this.

1.2.3.2 Histone methylation

Unlike DNA methylation, histone methylation is more complex and can activate or repress gene expression depending on where the modification occurs. Generally, lysine (K) or arginine (R) residues on H3 are methylated, although tails of other histones can also host the modification. The complexity of histone methylation is also caused by the number of methyl groups that are added to the histone tail. Arginine residues can host up to two methyl groups, while lysine residues can have up to three methyl groups, thus producing a mono- (me1), di- (me2) or tri-methylation (me3) status. Because arginine methylation remains poorly understood compared to lysine methylation, we will focus on the latter.

Table 2 A summary of common histone marks (Zhao and Garcia, 2015)

Histone modifications	Enyzyme	Function	Genomic location
H2BK120ub1	RNF20, RNF40	Activation	Gene body
H3K4me1	KMT2 family	Activation	Enhancer
H3K4me3	KMT2 family	Activation	Promoter
H3K9ac	GCN5	Activation	Promoter, Enhancer
H3K9me3	KMT1A, KMT1E	Represseion	Heterochromatin
H3K27ac	CBP, P300	Activation	Promoter, Enhancer
H3K27me3	EZH2	Repression	Promoter, Gene body
H3K36me3	KMT3A, KMT3B	Activation	Gene body
H3K36ac	GCN5	Activation	Promoter
H3K79me2/3	DOT1L	Activation	Gene body
H4K5ac	p300	Activation	Promoter, Enhancer
H4K8ac	p300	Activation	Promoter, Enhancer
H4K12ac	HAT1	Activation	Promoter, Enhancer

As several different lysine residues on various histones can be methylated (Table 2), there are also various respective enzymes that add or remove this modification from different sites. Methylations on H3K9 and H3K27 are thought to repress gene expression, whereas methylations on H3K4, H3K36 and H3K79 signal active transcription. In the case of the transcriptionally repressive mark, H3K27me3, the enzyme responsible for methylation is EZH2 (Enhancer of Zeste Homolog 2), a component of the PRC2 (Polycomb Repressive Complex 2) complex (Pirrotta, 1998). KDM6A (Lysine Demethylase 6A, also known as UTX), KDM6B (Lysine Demethylase 6B, also called JMJD3) and KDM6C (Lysine Demethylase 6C, as known as UTY, with relatively low activity), in turn, demethylate H3K27me2 and H3K27me3 (Agger et al., 2007; Walport et al., 2014). One "reader" of H3K27me3 is EED (Embryonic Ectoderm Development), a member of the PRC2 complex. The binding of EED to H3K27me3 leads to the spreading of the latter to nearby regions, ensuring the repressed status of the H3K27me3-marked region (Margueron et al., 2009). In the case of H3K4 methylation, the "writer" protein contains a SET-domain, which catalyzes the methylation of H3K4. In humans, there are six homologs that catalyze such reaction: SETD1A, SETD1B, MLL1, MLL2, MLL3 and MLL4 also known as KMT2F (Lysine Methyltransferase 2F), KMT2G (Lysine Methyltransferase 2G), KMT2A (Lysine Methyltransferase 2A), KMT2B (Lysine Methyltransferase 2B), KMT2C (Lysine Methyltransferase 2C) and KMT2D (Lysine Methyltransferase 2D), respectively (Shilatifard, 2012). The specificity of these methyltransferases is determined by their interacting partner, meaning associating with different interacting partners can change their catalytic activity (e.g. from catalyzing me1 to catalyzing both me1 and me2) (Patel et al., 2009). The "eraser", LSD1, also known as KDM1A (Lysine Demethylase 1A), was the first H3K4 demethylase identified (Shi et al., 2004) and KDM1A and its close homolog KDM1B (Lysine Demethylase 1B) both demethylate H3K4 (Ciccone et al., 2009). Apart from these two, JARID1 (Jumonji AT-rich Interactive Domain 1) family proteins, including JARID1A (Jumonji AT-rich Interactive Domain 1A), JARID1B (Jumonji AT-rich Interactive Domain 1B), JARID1C (Jumonji AT-rich Interactive Domain 1C) and JARID1D (Jumonji AT-rich Interactive Domain 1D), also have demethylating activity (Højfeldt et al., 2013). There are a few domains that are known to "read" histone methylation, such as PHD (Plant Homeodomain) domains, chromodomains, PWWP (Pro-Trp-Trp-Pro) domains, MBT (Malignant Brain Tumor) domains and WD40 domains (Yun et al., 2011).

Regarding its localization in the genome, H3K4me1 is often present at enhancer regions, distal regulatory elements, and has been widely used as a marker to predict such regulatory elements (Heintzman et al., 2007). Unlike H3K4me1, H3K4me3 is a marker for transcription start sites (TSSs) of actively transcribed genes (Santos-Rosa et al., 2002). These modifications are very informative for characterizing genomic loci and ENCODE (Encyclopedia of DNA Elements Project: also carried out numerous ChIP-seq (chromatin immunoprecipitation followed by sequencing) studies on these two histone marks.

As histone methylation has been shown to have an impact on many cellular processes (Greer and Shi, 2012), it is not surprising that histone methylation is often dysregulated in cancer. For example, translocations of KMT2A are present in 70% of infant leukemia patients and in other mixed-lineage leukemia patients to a lesser extent (Tenney and Shilatifard, 2005). As mentioned previously, more than 15% of ESCC patients have mutations in *KMT2D* and nearly 20% patients have mutations in *KDM6A* (Fig. 3). These mutations will directly affect the genome-wide H3K4 and H3K27 methylation landscapes, respectively, which can lead to altered gene expression. For instance, decreased H3K4me1 caused by KMT2D mutations and increased H3K27me3 caused by KDM6A mutation could collectively promote tumor progression, for example, by silencing tumor suppressor genes. Therefore, it is important to study the downstream effects caused by these mutations to determine whether they can be directly targeted, emerging as new cancer therapeutic options.

1.2.3.3 Histone acetylation

Acetylation of lysine residues on histones was first reported in 1964 and it was shown to potentially differentially regulate RNA (ribonucleic acid) production, transcription, at different genomic loci (Allfrey et al., 1964). Since then, there have been many advances in this field such as the identification of histone acetylation "writers" - histone acetyltransferases (HATs), histone acetylation "erasers" - histone deacetylases (HDACs) and histone acetylation "readers" – bromodomain (BD)-containing proteins (Fig. 10).

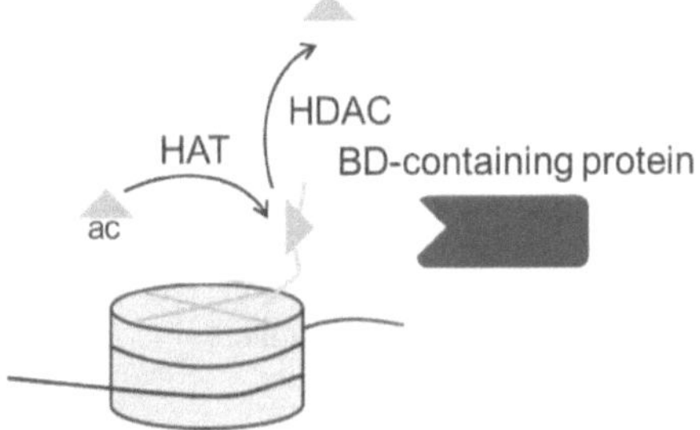

Fig. 10 Scheme showing the function of HATs, HDACs and BD-containing proteins. HATs catalyze the transfer of an acetyl group to the histone tail; HDACs remove the acetyl group from the acetylated residue; BD-containing proteins recognize acetylated lysine and regulate gene expression as well as chromatin accessibility.

Unlike histone methylation, histone acetylation neutralizes the otherwise positive charge of lysine residues, thus weakening the interaction between DNA and histone cores (Garcia-Ramirez et al., 1995; Tse et al., 1998), which can ultimately affect gene transcription. Common acetylation marks are summarized in Table 2.

1.2.3.3.1 Histone acetyltransferases

Histone acetylation is a process during which an acetyl group from the cofactor acetyl-CoA (coenzyme A) is transferred to a histone lysine residue. This reaction is catalyzed by HATs which comprise five major subfamilies – HAT1 (Histone Acetyltransferase 1), Gcn5/PCAF, MYST, p300/CBP and Rtt109 (specific for yeast) (Marmorstein and Zhou, 2014). Gcn5/PCAF were among the first histone transferases found (Brownell et al., 1996; Kleff et al., 1995). Crystal structure studies revealed that the acetylation activity of Gcn5 and PCAF is dependent on a core glutamate residue which serves as a base for catalysis (Tanner et al., 2000; Trievel et al., 1999). A similar active site structure was also discovered in the MYST protein family. In this case, a highly conserved glutamate residue was found in the MYST yeast homolog, Esa1, which upon mutation lead to diminished acetyltransferase activity (Yan et al., 2000). Unlike these two HAT families, p300 does not rely on glutamate residues for catalysis, but rather has two residues, Tyr1467 and Trp1436, which are conserved across p300/CBP family members. For p300, the mutation of these two residues significantly decreased its catalytic activity (Liu et al., 2008b). The difference in the active site residues in different HATs indicated that they could have different reaction mechanisms. Indeed, p300 was shown to use a "hit-and-run" mechanism which was distinct from Gcn5/PCAF and

MYST families (Zhang et al., 2014). It is also worth noting that the same HAT could use different catalyzing mechanisms when cooperating with different factors (Berndsen et al., 2007). Because HATs can function in different complexes, it is not surprising that they have substrate specificities. For example, GCN5/PCAF family, especially when associated with Spt-Ada-Gcn5 acetyltransferase complex (SAGA), have a preference for H3 (Nagy et al., 2010), while some MYST HATs only use H4 as substrate (Cai et al., 2010).

1.2.3.3.2 Histone deacetylases

Histone deacetylation, the removal of an acetyl group from histones, is realized by HDACs. There are 18 HDACs which can be further classified into four groups based on sequence homology: HDAC Class I, Class II, Class III and Class IV. Class I, II and III are similar to yeast Rpd3, Hda1 and Sir2, respectively. Class IV share similarities with Class I and II. Furthermore, HDACs are dependent on two distinct co-factors for catalyzing histone deacetylation (Table 3).

Table 3 HDAC classification system

Classes	Members	Dependency
Class I	HDAC1, HDAC2, HDAC3, HDAC8	Zinc ions
Class II	HDAC4, HDAC5, HDAC6, HDAC7, HDAC9, HDAC10	Zinc ions
Class III	SIRT1, SIRT2, SIRT3, SIRT4, SIRT5, SIRT6, SIRT7	NAD^+
Class IV	HDAC11	Zinc ions

Class I, II and IV HDACs are metalloenzymes, which rely on zinc ions for their catalytic activity (Seto and Yoshida, 2014). In fact, the deacetylation activity of HDAC8 was abolished when mutating histidine 142 (His142) and consequently preventing the chelation of the zinc ion in HDAC8 (Gantt et al., 2010). In contrast to other HDACs, class III HDACs rely on the cofactor NAD^+ (nicotinamide adenine dinucleotide) to deacetylate histones (Imai et al., 2000). Structural studies of class III HDACs have navigated the catalytic domain which is formed at the interface between a zinc-binding domain and the NDA^+-binding domain (Finnin et al., 2001). The substrate specificity of HDACs is more ambiguous compared with that of HATs. One big hurdle is that purified HDACs often lose their activity, so measuring their substrate specificity becomes very difficult (Seto and Yoshida, 2014). Besides that, the functional redundancy of HDAC family members also represent as a big obstacle for understanding the substrate specificity of a single HDAC. However, there are a few studies showing the substrate specificity of some HDACs. Using purified nucleosomes and HDAC3 complexes purified by immunoprecipitation (IP), HDAC3 complexes showed higher specificity for H2A, H4K5 and H4K12 compared to other substrates such as H4K8 and H4K16 (Johnson et al., 2002). Of note is that the results described above were based on HDAC3 immunocomplexes, such that the purity of the complex would directly affect the result. Given that HDAC inhibition has been and is being tested in clinical trials, it would be extremely helpful to understand HDAC substrate specificity.

1.2.3.3.3 Bromodomain-containing proteins

Acetylated lysine is recognized by BD-containing protein families, which comprise 46 BD-containing proteins. In total, these BD-containing proteins contain 61 bromodomains meaning that they comprise different numbers of bromodomains (one, two or multiple) (Filippakopoulos et al., 2012). These bromodomains can be classified into eight groups and each of them share over 30% sequence identity (Marmorstein and Zhou, 2014). Of those 46 BD-containing proteins, there are 11 proteins with two bromodomains and bromodomain and extra-terminal proteins (BETs) are important members of this group of proteins (Sanchez and Zhou, 2009).

The unraveling of the structure of bromodomains provided a mechanism explaining the recognition of acetylated lysine. Bromodomains are ~110 amino acids in length and consist of four left-handed α-helixes (αZ, αA, αB and αC) and two loops: ZA and BC. The ZA loop connects the αZ and αA helixes and the BC loop connects the αB and αC helixes. The interconnected α-helixes (ZA and BC) can then form a hydrophobic pocket which serves as the accommodating site for the acetylated lysine (Dhalluin et al., 1999). Several highly conserved residues in the ZA and BC loops were found important for the interaction between the acetylated lysine and the bromodomain (Sanchez and Zhou, 2009).

Further analysis also revealed that, in the case of BET proteins, neighboring histone modifications can influence the binding specify bromodomains. Filippakopoulos *et al.* did a massive screening to comprehensively determine the substrate specificity of human bromodomains. They found that the neighboring posttranslational modifications strongly affect the binding to acetylated lysine residues and that diacetylated H4 (especially at K5K8) is the preferred target of BET proteins (Filippakopoulos et al., 2012). The structural analysis of bromodomains also prompted the development of bromodomains inhibitors.

BET proteins comprise four members: BRD2 (Bromodomain-containing Protein 2), BRD3 (Bromodomain-containing Protein 3), BRD4 (Bromodomain-containing Protein 4) and BRDT (Bromodomain Testis-specific Protein). While BRD2, BRD3 and BRD4 are ubiquitously expressed, BRDT is exclusively expressed in testes indicating its role in spermatogenesis (Fig. 11), a process describing the development of sperms from spermatogonial stem cells.

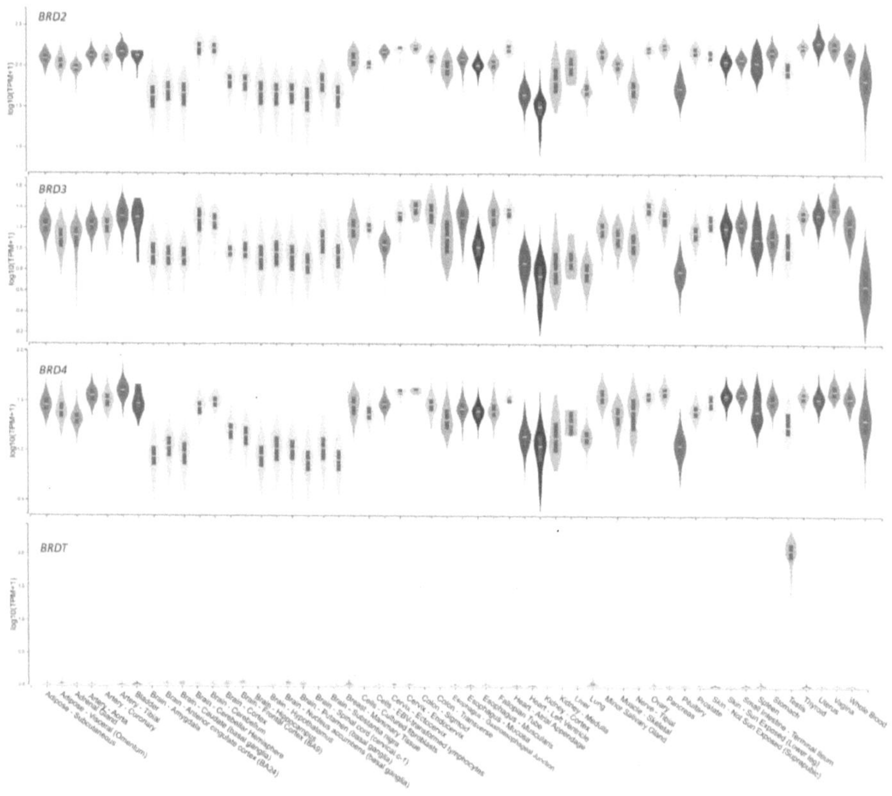

Fig. 11 Expression of *BRD2*, *BRD3*, *BRD4* and *BRDT* in normal tissues/organs. Y-axis: log10 transformed TPM (transcripts per million) + 1; X-axis: tissues/organs. (Data source: ____________________

Furthermore, BET proteins contain two tandem bromodomains, an extra-terminal (ET) domain and, in some cases, a C-terminal domain (CTD) as shown in Fig. 12. As aforementioned, bromodomains recognize acetylated lysine residues of histones (Dhalluin et al., 1999). It is also worth noting that bromodomains can recognize acetylated lysine residues of non-histone proteins such as GATA-binding protein 1 (GATA1, by BRD3) (Lamonica et al., 2011) and RelA (by BRD4) (Huang et al., 2009). The function of the ET domain is poorly understood compared to BDs, but recently a study showed that the ET domain can interact with other proteins such as NSD3 (Nuclear Receptor Binding SET Domain Protein 3) to activate transcription (Rahman et al., 2011). The CTD domain has been shown to interact with factors essential for transcription elongation, thus having a transcription activating role (Moon et al., 2005; Yang et al., 2005). Taken together, this suggests the critical role of BET proteins in transcription and gene regulation, which will be further described in the sections below.

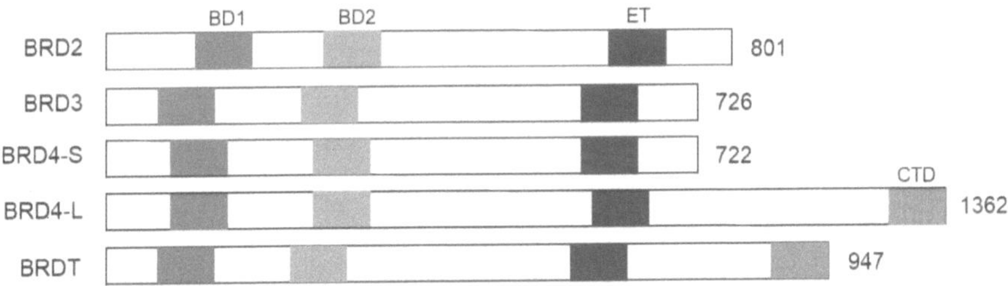

Fig. 12 Scheme showing the domains of BET family members. BRD4 has two major isoforms: BRD4-short (S) and BRD4-long (L). BD1: first bromodomain; BD2: second bromodomain; ET: extra-terminal domain; CTD: C-terminal domain.

There are many different histone acetylation marks, but can each of them be recognized by any bromodomain-containing proteins? Is there any specificity? There were already studies showing that BRD2 has higher affinity for H4K12ac of diacetylated H4K5acK12ac compared to monoacetylated H4K12ac (Huang et al., 2007; Umehara et al., 2010). To systematically answer this question, Filippakopoulos *et al.* did a massive screening to comprehensively determine the substrate specificity of human bromodomains. They found that the neighboring posttranslational modifications strongly affects the recognition and diacetylated H4 (especially at K5 and K8) is the preferred target for BET proteins(Filippakopoulos et al., 2012). However, these results were based on biochemical studies, and the binding affinity may be different under the physiological condition.

1.2.4 Histone acetylation in transcription and beyond

As previously described, histone acetylation is often associated with active transcription and different acetylation marks occupy various gene regulatory regions in the genome. Furthermore, the acetylation of histones can neutralize the charge of lysine residues (Garcia-Ramirez et al., 1995; Tse et al., 1998), likely affecting chromatin accessibility and ultimately gene transcription. Several mouse models with mutation or deletion of multiple factors involved in histone acetylation showed severe development defects or embryonic lethality (Montgomery et al., 2007; Shang et al., 2009; Tanaka et al., 2000), indicating the essential role of histone acetylation in development. In this section, we describe how multiple factors involved in histone acetylation can directly or indirectly interact with the transcription machinery to regulate gene expression. We further describe the possible advantages of targeting these factors in cancer.

1.2.4.1 HATs and HDACs

HATs and HDACs are two major families responsible for the balance of histone acetylation and can affect gene transcription in a histone-dependent or histone-independent manner. Firstly, histone acetylation can neutralize the lysine residues of histone tails and thus weaken the interaction between DNA and histones, leading to a more relaxed chromatin. The relaxed chromatin becomes more accessible to TFs, which can induce gene expression at affected loci (Zhao and Garcia, 2015).

But how is specificity determined? In the case of HATs, they can interact with other TFs to induce gene expression. For example, p300/CBP was regarded as a transcription coactivator before its acetyltransferase activity was found (Ogryzko et al., 1996). Typically, p300/CBP does not directly bind to DNA but is rather recruited to chromatin by other TFs with DNA-binding affinity, such as c-Jun (Arias et al., 1994; Bannister et al., 1995), CREB (Chrivia et al., 1993) and MyoD (Yuan et al., 1996). These DNA-binding TFs have a clear binding preference which can direct the association of HATs to specific genomic loci. Similarly, by the incorporation into a larger complex which contain other DNA-binding proteins, HDACs can be recruited to chromatin to deacetylate acetylysines leading the change of charge and compaction of chromatin. For example, the deacetylation of H4K16ac was shown to lead to DNA compaction and the assembly of striking senescence-associated heterochromatin foci (Contrepois et al., 2012).

The second way for HATs and HDACs to regulate transcription is through interacting with or directly modifying other factors. More specifically, HATs can acetylate non-histone proteins such as p53 (Gu and Roeder, 1997) and GATA1 (Boyes et al., 1998). The acetylation of these TFs can enhance their DNA-binding activity so that transcription is enhanced. However, if the acetylation site falls in the DNA-binding domain, it can disrupt the TF's DNA-binding affinity. For instance, the acetylation of Lys65 of high mobility group protein HMG-I/HMG-Y (HMGI(Y)) destabilizes the enhanceosome whereas acetylation of Lys71 can enhance the enhanceosome (Munshi et al., 2001).

Because HATs and HDACs can regulate gene expression in a refined manner, it is not hard to imagine that the deregulation of them would contribute to the development of diseases such as cancer. As previously mentioned, HATs can acetylate and potentially stabilize p53 enhancing its binding to its target genes and strengthening its tumor suppressive function (Liu et al., 1999). Consistently, HDAC inhibition can restore the acetylated p53 level and induce the expression of p21 (Zhao et al., 2006a). It is then not surprising that HATs are mutated in many cancers, such as p300 in ESCC (Gao et al., 2014). It is difficult to directly use HATs for clinical intervention for cancer treatment, but the inhibition of HDACs can increase acetylation levels which would be equivalent to stimulating HAT activity with regards to its histone acetyltransferase activity. In this case, the substrate specificity can still be an issue, because some specific acetylation can only be achieved by certain acetyltransferases. In other words, the specific antitumor acetylation mark catalyzed by a specific HAT might not be catalyzed by other HATs and the inhibition of HDACs cannot restore an acetylation which did not exist before. Nonetheless, employing HDAC inhibitors for treating cancer has yielded some success with many ongoing clinical trials and the FDA approval of HDAC inhibitors for treating certain types of lymphoma (Mann et al., 2007) and myeloma (Richardson et al., 2015).

1.2.4.2 BRD2 and BRD3

BET proteins, histone acetylation "readers", are also known to play a crucial role in transcription. When first identified, BRD2 was first characterized as a nuclear non-canonical protein kinase (Denis et al., 2000). Its transcription regulatory role was established later when its histone acetylation "reader" function was discovered. BRD2 can recognize acetylated histone tails, preferentially H4 tails, and subsequently recruit other transcription regulators including E2F factors (Peng et al., 2007), HATs (Sinha et al., 2005), chromatin remodelers (Denis et al., 2006) and subunits of the mediator complex (Jiang et al., 1998). The factors recruited by BRD2 can either alter chromatin accessibility or directly regulate the transcription machinery. Given the broad spectrum of BRD2-interacting partners, BRD2 is important for many cellular processes such as cell cycle. BRD2, along with BRD3, recognizes H4ac-rich region and allows RNA polymerase II (RNA Pol II) to transcribe through nucleosomes. Furthermore, the histone chaperone role of BRD2 is required for the expression of CycD1 (LeRoy et al., 2008), an important factor pushing cells from G1 to S phase. It has also been shown that the depletion of BRD2 significantly slowed the proliferation of embryonic fibroblast cells, thus playing an essential role in mouse embryonic development (Shang et al., 2009).

BRD3, like BRD2, can also interact with multiple chromatin remodeling complexes to modulate chromatin accessibility. More specifically, the ET domain of BRD3 can recognize a "KIKL" motif which is conserved among several chromatin remodeling complexes, such as BAF (BRG1/BRM Associated Factor), NuRD (Nucleosome Remodeling Deacetylase) and INO80 complexes (Wai et al., 2018). More surprisingly, the same motif can also be found in some transcriptional regulators such as AF9 and ENL, which are part of the super elongation complex (SEC) (Yokoyama et al., 2010), suggesting that BRD3 can act via AF9/ENL to regulate transcription elongation (Wai et al., 2018). BRD3 can also bind to acetylated GATA1, a hematopoietic transcription factor, and GATA1 can recruit BRD3 to chromatin seemingly independent of histone acetylation. Inhibiting the BRD3-GATA1 interaction, dissociates both of them from chromatin and interrupts erythroid maturation (Lamonica et al., 2011). Furthermore, fusions of BRD3 (or BRD4) with nuclear protein in testis (NUT) can provide growth advantage, contributing to the carcinogenesis of NUT midline carcinoma (NMC), an extremely aggressive malignancy (French et al., 2008). Thus, BRD2 and BRD3 interact with several transcription regulators, playing important roles in gene regulation, while controlling diverse cellular processes.

1.2.4.3 BRD4 and BRDT

BRD4 and BRDT are both comprised of two bromodomains, one ET domain and a CTD, an important domain for interactions with other proteins and complexes. The similarity in their domain composition indicates that BRD4 and BRDT might be functionally redundant. Still, BRDT is likely to have some unique functions because of its restricted expression in testes. As the most well-studied BET family member, BRD4 has been shown to be a critical player in transcription. BRD4 recognizes acetylated histones at promoters and enhancers via its bromodomains thus regulating gene expression (Filippakopoulos and Knapp, 2012; Mujtaba et al., 2007).

Enhancers are regulatory elements, which are often located in gene distal regions and, to a less extent, within genes bodies. Active enhancers are typically marked by several histone modification marks including H3K27ac and H3K4me1 (Creyghton et al., 2010; Heintzman et al., 2009). The existence of enhancers is another layer of the transcriptional regulatory network ensuring the right spatiotemporal gene expression program required by distinctive cell types. There are many more enhancers than coding genes in the human genome (Consortium et al., 2012), adding a lot more flexibility to the regulatory network for development, stress response, etc. Because they are typically situated in genomic regions far away from genes, they form a loop engaging the promoter of target gene and other transcriptional coactivators such as BET proteins, mediator complexes and HATs (Furlong and Levine, 2018; Schoenfelder et al., 2015). These enhancer-promoter loops bring the promoter and enhancer loci in close proximity together with TFs and other necessary transcription regulators, thus enabling enhancers to control their distant target genes.

Super enhancers (SEs) were identified much later by Richard Young and his colleagues (Hnisz et al., 2013; Whyte et al., 2013). By definition, SEs are long stretches of genomic loci containing multiple enhancers and they typically control target genes which are important for cell identity and lineage specification. SEs are often co-occupied by master TFs, cofactors and chromatin regulators, presenting very high transcriptional activity. Several studies have reported the output of the transcriptional activity of SEs in the form of enhancer RNAs (eRNAs) and their role in enhancer activity (Li et al., 2013; Mousavi et al., 2013). More recently, some studies tried to explain the strong transcriptional output associated with SEs by a more biophysical model termed "Phase separation" (Hahn, 2018; Sabari et al., 2018). In this model, a genomic locus with high concentration of TFs, coactivators and mediator complexes can go through liquid-liquid phase transition to form a phase-separated condensate with high transcriptional activity (Fig. 13). This way a particularly high concentration of a specific repertoire of factors is provided mainly to cell identity genes meeting their high transcriptional demand. Potentially, this type of condensates could also serve as a transcriptional hub for genes which require a similar set of TFs. Given the strong transcriptional activity and important role in development, it is not surprising that cancer cells hijack them for carcinogenesis (Hnisz et al., 2013; Whyte et al., 2013).

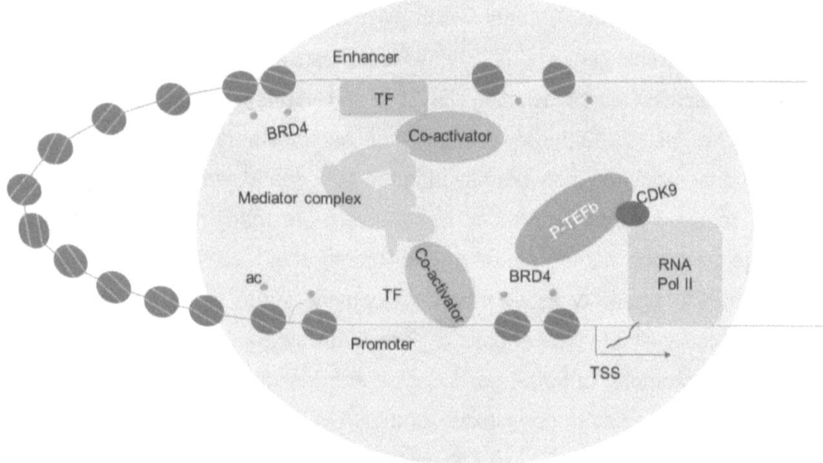

Fig. 13 A model showing a phase separated condensate containing SE and its interacting promoter region with several transcriptional regulators. The light green oval represents the phase separated condensate. TF: transcription factor; P-TEFb: positive transcription elongfation factor b.

BRD4 has been shown to mediate phase separation and disrupting the phase separation can lead to the dissociation of BRD4 from chromatin and potentially the disassembly of the phase-separated condensate (Sabari et al., 2018). The CTD domain of BRD4 exhibits a high content of serine residues, which gives rise to an intrinsically disordered domain promoting the formation of the liquid-liquid droplet phase separation. Similarly, RNA Pol II also has a serine-rich CTD which can facilitate the phase separation process (Boehning et al., 2018).

Apart from phase separation, BRD4 can also regulate transcription by interacting with P-TEFb (Positive Transcription Elongation Factor b), a complex comprising Cyclin T1 (CycT1) and CDK9 (Cyclin-Dependent Kinase 9). Upon the interaction of BRD4 with P-TEFb, CDK9 phosphorylates the CTD domain of RNA Pol II, which then leads to the release of RNA Pol II from the promoter region allowing for transcriptional elongation. The knock-down of BRD4 leads to decreased phosphorylation of the CTD of RNA Pol II and lower transcriptional activity, suggesting that BRD4 is a positive transcription regulator (Moon et al., 2005; Yang et al., 2005). Besides, there are also studies showing that BRD4 has kinase activity which enables BRD4 to directly phosphorylate the CTD of RNA Pol II at Ser2, and that this process can be blocked by pharmacologically inhibiting BRD4 (Devaiah et al., 2012).

BRDT is a close paralog to BRD4 that is only expressed in testes and has been studied mostly in spermatogenesis. Given the role of BRD4 in transcription elongation, it is reasonable to postulate that BRDT also regulates transcription through the interaction with P-TEFb. Indeed, the interaction between BRDT and CycT1/CDK9 was confirmed in spermatogenic cells. Furthermore, the depletion of Brdt in mice decreased the expression of more than 2000 genes, suggesting its role in transcription regulation. Moreover, ChIP-seq of BRDT in spermatocytes uncovered that BRDT specifically binds to promoters of testis-specific genes which are important for meiosis (Gaucher et al., 2012). However, because of its testis-specific expression, the role of BRDT in transcription regulation is likely underexplored.

To date, BRDT is best characterized for its role in chromatin remodeling during spermatogenesis. During this process, BRDT aids in the histone-to-protamine transition, which allows for massive chromatin compaction in post-meiotic cells. Protamines are a type of arginine-rich nuclear protein, which are smaller than histones in size (4.5 kilo Dalton vs 15 kilo Dalton). The histone-to-protamine transition consists of substituting histones by protamines, allowing for a denser chromatin compaction, which also makes the chromatin more resistant to mutation. Mice carrying a BD1-lacking Brdt can develop normally until the histone-to-protamine exchange, indicating that BD1 is crucial for histone-to-protamine transition but dispensable for the meiotic gene program (Gaucher et al., 2012). Because the histone-to-protamine transition involves nearly the whole genome, there has to be signal to trigger this process. Indeed, right before the histone-to-protamine transition, a genome-wide hyperacetylation was observed in multiple species (Hazzouri et al., 2000; Meistrich et al., 1992). Subsequently, BRDT can recognize that hyperacetylation signal to initiate the histone-to-protamine transition. Furthermore, the ectopic expression of Brdt in somatic cells can induce a large-scale genome rearrangement upon histone hyperacetylation induced by trichostatin A (TSA), an HDAC inhibitor. Moreover, this chromatin-remodeling function of BRDT has been shown to be dependent on both BDs and their flanking region (Pivot-Pajot et al., 2003). Another study showed that BRDT can not only bind to acetylated histone but also to DNA via its BD1. The binding of BRDT to DNA is non-specific but can facilitate the histone-BRDT interaction (Miller et al., 2016). This is probably essential for the massive and quick genome-wide histone-to-protamine transition.

1.2.4.4 Targeting histone acetylation "readers" in cancer

Given the important role of BET proteins in gene regulation and the fact that BET proteins have been found to be dysregulated in several cancers, BET inhibition represents an attractive target for cancer treatment. NUT midline carcinoma (NMC) is a rare but extremely aggressive malignancy with a median survival of six to seven months (French, 2010). Interestingly, 75% of NMC patients display a gene fusion event in which most of the coding region of *NUT* was fused with *BRD4* or *BRD3*, creating a chimeric gene (French, 2010; Miyoshi et al., 2001). The fused BRD-NUT protein has been shown to block differentiation and to confer proliferation advantages, thus representing an attractive therapeutic target.

In fact, initial studies of BET inhibition in NMC have shown promising results. JQ1, a BET protein small molecule inhibitor, can bind to both bromodomains of all BET proteins to abolish its BD-dependent transcriptional regulation (Fig. 14) (Filippakopoulos et al., 2010). This inhibitor was shown to compete with the acetyl group of histones, the natural substrate of BETs and the BRD-NUT oncoprotein. This competition led to the dissociation of BRD-NUT oncoprotein from chromatin, promoting the differentiation of NMC cells. Moreover, low dose JQ1 treatment could also induce cell cycle arrest at G1 phase in NMC cells. This was confirmed again in a patient-derived xenograft model, showing the potency of this BET protein small molecule inhibitor (Filippakopoulos et al., 2010). Since then, many pharmaceutical companies have developed multiple BET inhibitors, such as iBET762 (GSK) and OTX015 (Merck). These inhibitors have been or are being tested in clinical trials to fully understand their antitumor efficacy. Results from NMC and hematologic cancer are not extremely good, but encouraging and more clinical trials in solid tumors are currently ongoing as reviewed by Belkina and Denis as well as by Stathis and Bertoni (Belkina and Denis, 2012; Stathis and Bertoni, 2018).

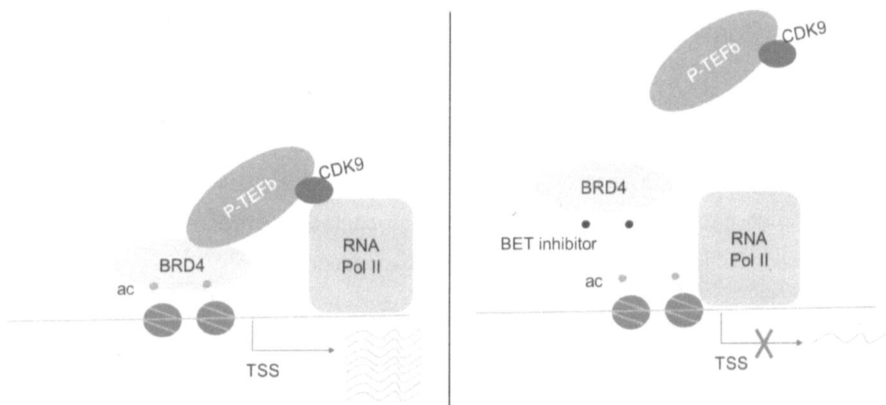

Fig. 14 Illustration of BET inhibition and its downstream effects on gene transcription. BRD4 can recognize acetylated histone at TSS and interact with P-TEFb which then phosphorylates RNA Pol II to promote transcription elongation. BET inhibitors can competitively bind to the bromodomain of BRD4 to disrupt its interaction with acetylated histone.

Notably, most of the BET inhibitors developed are pan-BET inhibitors meaning they target every BD of BRD2, BRD3, BRD4 and BRDT. However, different BDs within the same protein, such as BRDT (Gaucher et al., 2012), showed different function, which led to the idea of targeting a specific bromodomain. Recently, several BD-specific inhibitors were developed and indeed showed distinctive effects (Chiang, 2014; Gilan et al., 2020; Picaud et al., 2013). These aspects should also be taken into consideration for future designs of preclinical or clinical tests.

BET proteins also possess BD-independent functions, through the action of their ET domain and/or CTD, such that a BD-independent targeting of BET proteins may also be beneficial. However, it is challenging to directly target the ET or CTD domain of BET proteins, such that promoting the degradation of the entire protein may serve as an alternative. Proteolysis targeting chimeras (PROTACs) compounds are molecules which target a specific factor for degradation and have shown a great potential in the pharmacology field (Sun et al., 2019). Degradation of BET proteins has also been achieved using the PROTAC methodology and their anticancer effects have been shown in multiple cancer models (Raina et al., 2016; Shi et al., 2019; Winter et al., 2017; Zengerle et al., 2015; Zhang et al., 2020a). Given the promising results, these compounds should be further evaluated in preclinical models to estimate their anticancer potential.

1.2.5 Chromatin remodeling and the three-dimensional (3D) genome

Like DNA methylation and histone modification, chromatin remodeling can directly change the chromatin accessibility, thus exposing or burying certain chromatin fragments, leading to gene expression change. Likewise, the spatial organization of the human genome directly affects chromatin contact, such as enhancer-promoter interaction, which can result in altered gene expression.

1.2.5.1 Chromatin remodeling

Highly dynamic cellular process needs a dynamic chromatin structure for fine-tuning gene expression. Chromatin remodeler complexes are responsible for re-arranging the chromatin to maintain chromatin dynamics. There are four major chromatin remodeling families: switch/sucrose non-fermentable (SWI/SNF), imitation switch (ISWI), chromodomain helicase DNA-binding (CHD), and INO80 (Clapier et al., 2017). Their function involves many aspects of chromatin dynamics and can be summarized into three different points: nucleosome assembly, chromatin accessibility and nucleosome editing. Chromatin accessibility can be further classified into three: nucleosome sliding, nucleosome eviction and histone dimer eviction. All of the actions described above can affect gene expression and the deregulation of chromatin remodeling is common in cancer (Kaur et al., 2019; Nair and Kumar, 2012; Wolffe, 2001).

1.2.5.2 Deciphering 3D genome using HiC

The human genome is organized in a 3D manner involving a hierarchical packing of DNA and its associated factors. The higher order of genome organization is highly dynamic and possesses a spatiotemporal pattern. The appropriate folding of the genome can bring distal regulatory elements, such as enhancers, in proximity to their targets and segregate regulatory elements from non-target genes to avoid gene expression dysregulation. Artificially disrupting the higher order of genome organization can lead to abnormal folding of the genome, which ultimately influences the transcription of genes located in that region (Arzate-Mejía et al., 2020). Therefore, the 3D structure of the genome has been shown to contribute to development (Gorkin et al., 2014; Stadhouders et al., 2019; Zheng and Xie, 2019) and disease progression (Kantidze et al., 2020).

Given the importance of the 3D genome, it is critical to systematically study it using high-throughput methods. Chromatin conformation capture (3C) was developed to study the folding of chromosomes in yeast (Dekker et al., 2002). This method was designed to test the interaction between two known genomic loci. Cells were first fixed by formaldehyde and subsequently subjected to restriction enzyme digestion. Following, a ligation step was carried out to ligate two DNA ends. Finally, a quantitative real-time PCR (qPCR) was performed to detect the DNA contact. 4C (circularized 3C) (Simonis et al., 2006; Zhao et al., 2006b) and 5C (3C carbon copy) (Dostie et al., 2006) were developed to increase the throughput, however, they could still not achieve the goal of mapping the whole-genome wide DNA contacts. The development of HiC (Chromatin conformation capture followed by high-throughput sequencing) finally resolved issues regarding throughput by incorporating biotin-labeled dNTPs (deoxyribonucleotide triphosphates) (Lieberman-Aiden et al., 2009). Many other techniques with specific designs were then derived from HiC such as capture C (Hughes et al., 2014) and HiChIP (HiC followed by ChIP) (Mumbach et al., 2016). HiChIP utilizes one more IP step after ligating biotin-filled ends to select a subset of interactions which are coupled with the protein of interest (Fig. 15). This measure can dramatically enrich the targeted DNA contact thereby reducing the sequencing depth required for detecting DNA interactions.

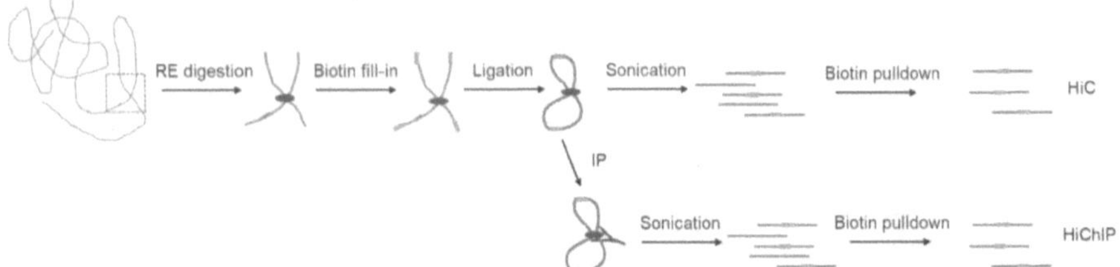

Fig. 15 A simplified scheme showing the workflow of HiC and HiChIP. Cells are first fixed and digested with a certain restriction enzyme (RE) to generate sticky ends which are filled by biotin-labeled deoxyribonucleotides (dNTPs). Sticky ends of interacting chromatin fragments are ligated. For HiC, ligated chromatin is decrosslinked and sheared before the biotin enrichment. As for HiChIP, an extra step of immunoprecipitation (IP) is utilized to enrich chromatin associated with the protein of interest and the following steps are identical to HiC.

1.3 Aims of this project

ESCC, the predominant subtype of esophageal cancer, is a common and deadly malignancy with an over-all 5-year survival rate of 15 – 20%. The incidence rate of ESCC is particularly high in certain geographic regions, such as East Asia. Over the last decades, advances in endoscopy have helped in the diagnosis and treatment of ESCC patients. However, those patients diagnosed at early stages only make up a small portion, as the majority of patients still need to undergo surgery in combination with chemotherapy/chemoradiotherapy. Precision oncology has been applied to and benefited certain groups of patients. Although there is a significant portion of ESCC patients with dysregulated EGFR signaling pathway, many clinical trials testing EGFR inhibitors have failed, which highlights the need for the identification of novel therapeutic targets. Recent genomic studies have shown many dysregulated epigenetic pathways in ESCC, implying that targeting certain epigenetic factors in ESCC may bring clinical benefits.

The goal of this study was to systematically screen epigenetic factors for novel therapeutic targets. Ideally, these therapeutic targets should be: 1. tissue-specific and 2. differentially expressed in ESCC patients. Meeting these criteria, the newly identified therapeutic target would minimize the side effects and help to stratify patients for the targeted therapy. Once we identified the therapeutic target, we planned to check its effects on cell proliferation and migration using siRNA-mediated knock-down or CRISPR/Cas9-mediated knock-out techniques. In order to uncover the underlying mechanism, we sought to utilize RNA-seq and ChIP-seq to identify pathways and/or factors that are related to the newly identified protein. After knowing the associated factor, we intended to explore the functional interplay between them by analyzing their target genes and genomic occupancy. In order to confirm the functional interplay between them, we aimed to experimentally test the impact of them on each other's gene signature. By analyzing the chromatin topology, we intended to test whether the function of the potential therapeutic target is mediated by long-range chromatin interaction. Furthermore, to examine the feasibility of targeting the newly identified protein, we planned to pharmacologically inhibit the target to mimic the effects of gene knockdown. With all that knowledge, we finally aimed at proposing new therapeutic targets for the treatment of ESCC.

Chapter 2: Manuscript

Bromodomain protein BRDT directs ΔNp63 function and super enhancer activity in a subset of esophageal squamous cell carcinomas

Xin Wang[1], Ana P Kutschat[1], Moyuru Yamada[2], Evangelos Prokakis[1], Patricia Böttcher[1], Koji Tanaka[2], Yuichiro Doki[2], Feda H. Hamdan[3], Steven A. Johnsen[1,3,*]

[1]Clinic for General, Visceral and Pediatric Surgery, University Medical Center Göttingen, Göttingen, 37077, Germany

[2]Department of Gastroenterological Surgery, Graduate School of Medicine, Osaka University, Osaka, 565-0871, Japan

[3]Gene Regulatory Mechanisms and Molecular Epigenetics Lab, Division of Gastroenterology and Hepatology, Mayo Clinic, Rochester, MN, 55905, USA

* To whom correspondence should be addressed. Tel: +1-507-255-6138; Fax: +1-507-255-6318;

2.2 BACKGROUND

Esophageal cancer is a common malignancy and the 6th leading cause of cancer-related deaths worldwide. The overall 5-year survival rate remains unchanged for the last few decades, ranging from 15% to 25% (Siegel et al., 2019). Esophageal cancer consists of two major histological subtypes – esophageal squamous cell carcinoma (ESCC) and esophageal adenocarcinoma (EAC). ESCC, the predominant histological subtype, accounts for 90% of esophageal cancer cases and shows an especially high incidence rate in certain geographical locations, such as East Asia (Smyth et al., 2017). Recently, large scale genomic and epigenomic studies have revealed the genetic and epigenetic landscape of ESCC and identified recurring mutations or deletions in *TP53*, *CDKN2A* and *RB1*, and frequent amplifications of *SOX2, TP63* and *FGFR1* (Smyth et al., 2017), making them essential parts of the molecular repertoire defining the "squamous" subtype. Notably, several epigenetic modulators including *CREBBP, EP300, KMT2C* and *KMT2D,* are also frequently mutated (Gao et al., 2014). While these studies have helped in the molecular characterization of ESCC, they have yet to lead to specific molecular targeted therapies for this particular subtype (Lin et al., 2018).

Epigenetic regulation is crucial for cells to integrate environmental stimuli and intrinsic regulatory networks and maintain cellular and tissue homeostasis. Furthermore, dysregulation of epigenetic regulatory mechanisms contributes to tumorigenesis, tumor progression and the acquisition of therapeutic resistance (Morel et al., 2020). However, in contrast to genetic alterations, epigenetic alterations are usually reversible, thereby providing an ideal possibility for therapeutic intervention. One family of epigenetic regulators that has emerged as a particularly effective and accessible therapeutic target are the Bromodomain and Extra-terminal (BET) family of epigenetic reader proteins. The BET family comprises BRD2, BRD3, BRD4 and BRDT, and functions by recognizing acetyl groups on both histones (Belkina and Denis, 2012) and non-histone proteins (Shi et al., 2014) via their tandem bromodomains. BRD4, the most well-studied BET protein, binds acetylated histones at promoters and enhancers of its target genes where it functions together with the Mediator complex and various other cofactors to promote productive transcriptional elongation by RNA Polymerase II (Moon et al., 2005). Notably, BRD4 enrichment is a hallmark of so-called super enhancers (SEs), long stretches of transcriptionally active chromatin regions displaying a particularly high density of transcription factors and cofactors, which are known to regulate key genes essential for cell identity specification and disease progression (Lovén et al., 2013; Sabari et al., 2018). Given the critical role in transcriptional regulation, BET proteins have been shown to play important roles in development, homeostasis and various diseases including cancer, thus emerging as novel therapeutic targets for cancer and other diseases (Dawson et al., 2012). While pan-BET inhibitors are being tested in clinical trials for several different malignancies including lymphoma, breast cancer and prostate cancer (Stathis and Bertoni, 2018), the biological understanding of the other BET family members BRD2, BRD3 and BRDT in cancer is still very limited.

The concept of precision medicine is based on the assumption that targeted therapies developed against specific cancer-relevant proteins may improve clinical outcome while helping to avoid non-specific adverse effects often caused by standard chemotherapies. Thus, highly specific small molecule inhibitors are being intensively investigated as the next generation of anti-cancer therapies (Sawyers, 2004). In the case of some malignancies such as breast cancer (Goutsouliak et al., 2020), lung cancer (Yuan et al., 2019) and leukemia (Kayser et al., 2017), such approaches have dramatically increased patient survival rates. However, despite extensive trials, successful targeted therapy options for ESCC remain limited (Okines et al., 2011). For example, various tyrosine receptor kinase inhibitors such as inhibitors against *EGFR*, which is often overexpressed in ESCC, have been tested in ESCC patients. Nevertheless, most have failed to improve survival and were accompanied to varying degrees by unwanted side effects (Dutton et al., 2014; Ilson et al., 2011), necessitating the identification of novel therapeutic targets with lower toxicity.

In this study, we sought to identify novel therapeutic targets from a comprehensive collection of epigenetic factors, which are tissue-specific and differentially expressed in ESCC. Surprisingly, the testis-specific BET family member, BRDT was identified as a putative target, being aberrantly expressed in over 30% of an ESCC cohort, while modulating the migratory potential of ESCC cells. Mechanistically, BRDT co-localizes and interacts with ΔNp63, a defining factor of the squamous subtype in cancer, and acts as a regulatory switch for ΔNp63-driven transcription activation. The aberrant expression of BRDT rewires and enhances the dependencies of ΔNp63, modulating the expression of super enhancer (SE) associated genes. In conclusion, we show that

BRDT is expressed in a subset of ESCC and enhances the ΔNp63-dependent transcriptional program to promote cell migration in ESCC.

2.3 RESULTS

2.3.1 Unbiased screening identified BRDT as a unique feature in a distinct subset of ESCC

Due to their reversible nature and potential targetability, epigenetic modulators represent ideal candidates for anti-cancer therapy. In order to uncover potential specific targets for ESCC treatment that would be predicted to elicit minimal side effects, we sought to identify targetable epigenetic regulators, which are tissue specific and differentially expressed in ESCC. In order to achieve this, we exploited publicly available expression data (Lin et al., 2018; Wells et al., 2015) and identified four genes – *PADI1, PADI3, BRDT, CTCFL* – which displayed high levels of tissue specificity and differential expression in ESCC (Fig. 16A, Additional file 2: Table S1). Given the potential targetability of BRDT by small molecule BET inhibitors, we further investigated this testis-specific member of the BET family of proteins. To date, most studies examined BRDT function in male germ cells (Gaucher et al., 2012; Matzuk et al., 2012; Miller et al., 2016; Pivot-Pajot et al., 2003; Shang et al., 2007), however, we found *BRDT* to be expressed in more than 30% of ESCC (Kim et al., 2017) (Additional file 3: Table S2). To more generally explore the expression pattern of BRDT in cancer, we leveraged data from The Cancer Genome Atlas (TCGA) consortium and observed that *BRDT* is significantly expressed in several malignancies in addition to esophageal cancer and testicular cancer, including breast, lung and head and neck cancers (Fig. 16B). We next investigated whether BRDT was preferentially expressed in a certain histological subtype of esophageal cancer and found *BRDT* to be preferentially expressed in ESCC (Fig. 16C, Additional file 3: Table S2). Notably, consistent with the TCGA data, we were able to confirm that *BRDT* is expressed in an independent cohort of ESCC compared to adjacent normal tissue (Fig. 16D). Moreover, using data from the Cancer Cell Line Encyclopedia (CCLE) (Barretina et al., 2012) we identified two BRDT-positive (KYSE180 and TE6) and two BRDT-negative ESCC cell lines (KYSE70 and KYSE150) and confirmed BRDT expression in KYSE180 and TE6 cells (Fig. 16E).

In order to examine potential tumorigenic functions of BRDT, we utilized CRISPR/Cas9-mediated genome editing and siRNA-mediated knockdown to efficiently deplete BRDT protein levels (Fig. 16E). While depletion of BRDT did not appreciably affect cell proliferation, migration potential was largely abolished, suggesting a role of BRDT in controlling cell migration (Fig. 16F, G, Additional file 1: Fig. S1A-C). Together, these results indicate that BRDT is aberrantly expressed in a subset of ESCC and may function to promote cell migration.

Fig. 1

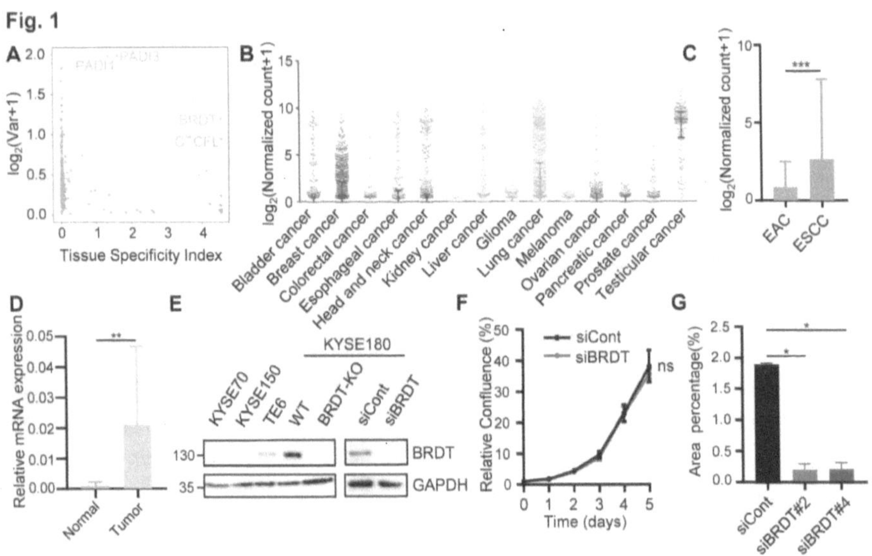

Fig. 1 Unbiased screening identifies BRDT as a potential therapeutic target for precision medicine in ESCC. (A) Scatter plot showing tissue specificity in normal tissues (y axis) and expression variance (x axis) of epigenetic factors in ESCC. (B) Expression of *BRDT* in different cancer entities. (C) Box plot showing 10-90 percentile of the expression of *BRDT* in different histological subtypes. Unpaired t-test was used. (D) Quantitative real-time PCR analysis of *BRDT* expression in tumor and adjacent normal tissues presented with box plot showing 10-90 percentile. Samples of 31 patients were evaluated. Paired t-test was used. *ACTB* was used to normalize gene expression. (E) Western blot analysis of BRDT in various ESCC cell lines and siRNA-mediated knock-down of BRDT and CRISPR/Cas9-mediated knock-out of BRDT in KYSE180 cells. (F) Growth kinetics analysis of control (siCont) and BRDT knock-down (siBRDT) in KYSE180. Data are represented as mean ± SD, n=4. Paired t-test was used. (G) Quantification of migrated cells upon BRDT knock-down with different siRNAs in KYSE180. Data are represented as mean ± SD, n=2. Unpaired t-test was used. ****: $P \leq 0.0001$, ***: $P \leq 0.005$, **: $P \leq 0.01$, *: $P \leq 0.05$, ns: not significant.

2.3.2 BRDT regulates gene expression programs related to cell migration in ESCC cells

In order to gain mechanistic insight into the role of BRDT in ESCC, we performed mRNA-seq upon depletion of BRDT in KYSE180 cells. As BET proteins generally function as transcriptional activators, we performed pathway enrichment analysis on genes down-regulated following BRDT depletion. This approach identified extracellular matrix (ECM) organization-related pathways (Fig. 17A), processes critical for cell migration (Gilkes et al., 2014; Hynes, 2014), as being key downstream targets of BRDT. RNA-seq analysis of a second BRDT-positive ESCC cell line (TE6) revealed a significant overlap between the regulated genes of two different cell lines (Fig. 17B, C) and could be validated by quantitative real-time PCR (qRT-PCR) analyses in both cell systems (Fig. 17D).

Since BET proteins bind to acetylated lysines and do not possess intrinsic sequence-specific DNA binding capacity, we sought to identify specific transcription and epigenetic regulatory factors associated with BRDT-associated transcriptional regulation. Strikingly, when examining transcription factors enriched on genes downregulated upon BRDT depletion, we identified TP63 as a top candidate (Fig. 17E). This finding is consistent with the TP63 isoform ΔNp63 being a key regulator of the squamous-specific transcriptional program (Hamdan and Johnsen, 2018; Moses et al., 2019; Smyth et al., 2017; Somerville et al., 2018). Consistently, gene set enrichment analysis (GSEA) also identified TP63-related gene signatures as being downregulated in BRDT-depleted KYSE180 and TE6 cells (Fig. 17F). These results uncover BRDT as a novel regulator of cell migration-related and ΔNp63-dependent gene programs in ESCC.

Fig. 2

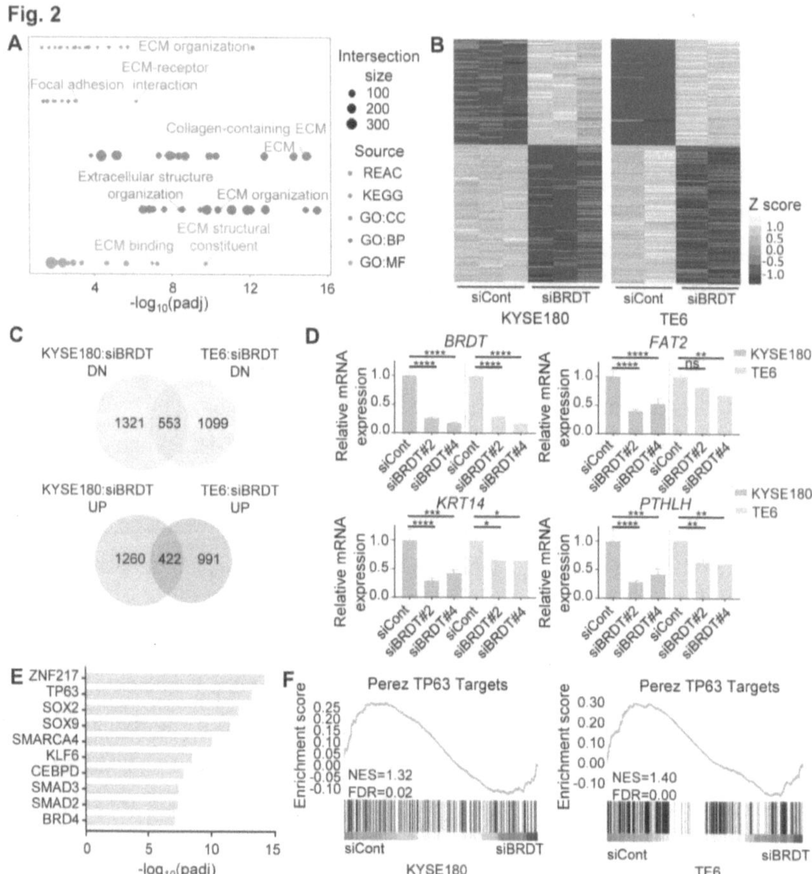

Fig. 2 Transcriptomic profiling reveals the role of BRDT in cell migration. (A) Pathway analysis of down-regulated genes upon BRDT knock-down in KYSE180. (B) Heatmaps showing the robustness of the RNA-seq data in KYSE180 (left) and TE6 (right). The commonly regulated (padj<0.05 and log2FC ≤ -0.5 or log2FC ≥ 0.5) genes of KYSE180 and TE6 are plotted. (C) Venn diagrams showing the overlap of significantly regulated (padj<0.05 and log2FC ≤ -0.5 or log2FC ≥ 0.5) genes between KYSE180 and TE6. (D) Quantitative real-time PCR validation of down-regulated genes upon BRDT knock-down in KYSE180 and TE6. GAPDH was used to normalize gene expression. Data are represented as mean ± SD, n=3. Unpaired one-way ANOVA test followed by Dunnett's test was used. ****: P≤0.0001, ***: P≤0.005, **: P≤0.01, *: P≤0.05, ns: not significant. (E) ChIP enrichment analysis (ChEA) showing enriched factors of commonly down-regulated genes between KYSE180 and TE6. (F) GSEA showing TP63 target genes are regulated by BRDT in KYSE180 and TE6.

2.3.3 BRDT occupies epigenetically active genomic regulatory regions

While BRDT occupancy was previously examined in germ cells (Gaucher et al., 2012), its role in gene regulation and genome occupancy has not been investigated in tumor cells to date. In order to dissect the function of BRDT in controlling gene expression in ESCC, we performed genome-wide chromatin immunoprecipitation-sequencing (ChIP-seq) analyses of BRDT in KYSE180 cells. These results revealed that BRDT is localized both to promoter proximal and distal enhancer regions in KYSE180 cells (Fig. 18A). Since BET proteins have a high-affinity towards diacetylated histone 4 (H4) tails (Filippakopoulos et al., 2012), we also performed epigenome mapping studies for several histone modifications. Specifically, we examined the occupancy of H4K5ac, H3K9ac, H3K27ac, H3K4me1, H3K4me3 and H3K27me3 in KYSE180 cells. We found that BRDT preferentially co-localizes with active histone marks such as H3K27ac, H3K9ac, H4K5ac, H3K4me1 and H3K4me3, further supporting a positive role for BRDT in regulating gene expression. Moreover, consistent with biophysical studies showing that murine BRDT has a binding preference for acetylated lysine 5 (K5) and lysine 8 (K8) on H4 (Morinière et al., 2009), we observed a higher concordance of BRDT occupancy with H4K5ac compared to either H3K27ac or H3K9ac (Fig. 18B). To gain more insight into the epigenomic context of BRDT occupancy, we classified the ESCC genome into different chromatin states based on the investigated histone marks (Fig. 18C) and quantified the overlap of BRDT-enriched regions with each defined state. This revealed that BRDT is mainly localized to active transcription start sites (TSSs) and enhancers (Fig. 18D, E), providing further support that BRDT is a positive transcriptional regulator.

In order to identify potential transcription factors directing BRDT activity in ESCC, we performed motif analyses on BRDT-enriched genomic regions. Consistent with the results of our transcriptome data, consensus motifs bound by TP63 were highly enriched in BRDT-occupied regions (Fig. 18F). Thus, these genome-wide occupancy studies illustrate that BRDT preferentially binds to active TSS and enhancers, and support a potential role in directing ΔNp63 activity in ESCC.

Fig. 3

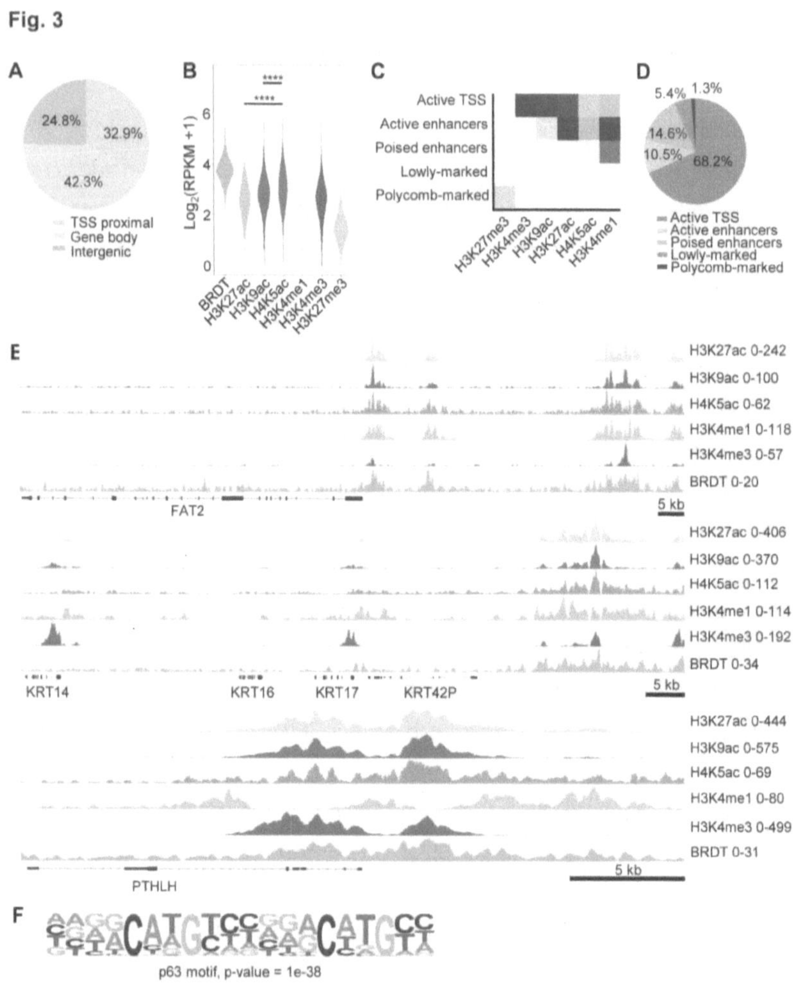

Fig. 3 ChIP-seq uncovers the genomic occupancy of BRDT in KYSE180. (A) Analysis of genomic occupancy of BRDT. (B) Violin plot showing the signal strength of BRDT on various histone modifications bound regions. Unpaired one-way ANOVA test followed by Dunnett's test was used. ****: P≤0.0001, ***: P≤0.005, **: P≤0.01, *: P≤0.05, ns: not significant. (C) ChromHMM analysis identifying different chromatin states based on histone marks. (D) Distribution of BRDT over different chromatin states. (E) ChIP-seq tracks of BRDT and other histone marks at FAT2, KRT14 and PTHLH loci. (F) Motif analysis of BRDT bound regions identifying p63 motif.

2.3.4 BRDT co-localizes with the squamous transcription factor ΔNp63

Given our findings that BRDT is required for the expression of a p63-controlled transcription program and an enrichment of a p63 binding motif in BRDT-occupied genomic regions, we hypothesized that BRDT and ΔNp63 may functionally and physically interact with one another. To address this, we performed ChIP-seq analysis for ΔNp63 in KYSE180 cells and examined its co-localization with BRDT. Strikingly, BRDT co-occupied many active ΔNp63-bound regions (i.e. ΔNp63-bound regions marked by H3K27ac) supporting a functional interplay between BRDT and ΔNp63 (Fig. 19A). Individual examples of genes co-occupied by BRDT and ΔNp63 included *KRT14*, *FAT2* and *PTHLH*, whose expression is ΔNp63-dependent and tightly associated with a squamous gene expression program (Fig. 19B). Based on the co-occupancy of ΔNp63 and BRDT we hypothesized that the two proteins may form a complex together. In order to test this, we performed co-immunoprecipitation (CoIP) analysis. Indeed, immunoprecipitation of BRDT resulted in a co-immunoprecipitation of ΔNp63 (Fig. 19C).

Given our initial finding that BRDT was required for the expression of published TP63-dependent genes and evidence of physical cooperation throughout the genome of ESCC cells, we next sought to validate the cooperative function of BRDT and ΔNp63 in ESCC by examining the effects of depleting ΔNp63 on transcription. Consistent with the notion that BRDT plays a central role in regulating ΔNp63 activity, we found an overlap between BRDT- and ΔNp63-dependent genes in both KYSE180 and TE6 cells (Fig. 19D). Exemplary, three genes co-occupied by BRDT and ΔNp63 (*FAT2*, *KRT14* and *PTHLH*), could be confirmed to be down-regulated upon depletion of either BRDT (Fig. 17D) or ΔNp63 (Fig. 19E). Given our previous observation that BRDT was required for KYSE180 cell migration, we hypothesized that depletion of either the responsible transcription factor providing sequence specificity to BRDT activity (ΔNp63) or a downstream ΔNp63/BRDT target previously shown to control cell migration in human squamous carcinoma cells (*FAT2*, (Matsui et al., 2008)), may phenocopy the effects of BRDT depletion on cell migration. Remarkably, we observed that the depletion of either ΔNp63 or FAT2 significantly decreased cell migration (Fig. 19F, Additional file 1: Fig. S2). Taken together, these results suggest that ΔNp63 physically interacts with and functionally cooperates with BRDT to transcriptionally activate genes essential for cell migration.

Fig. 4

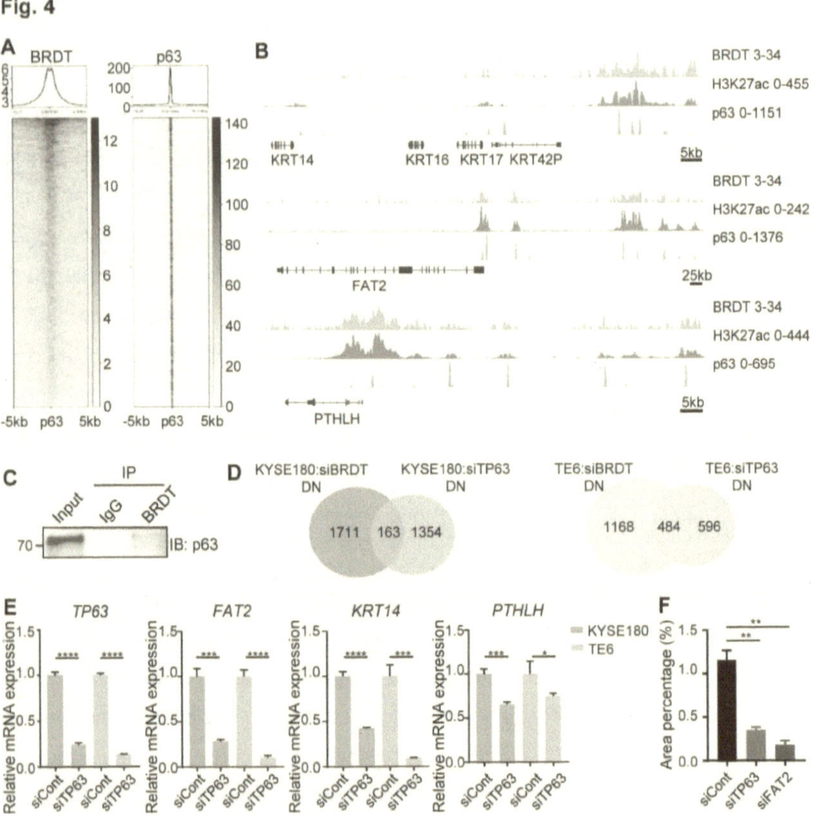

Fig. 4 BRDT co-localizes with the squamous transcription factor ΔNp63. (A) Heatmaps showing the co-occupancy of BRDT and p63. Plots are centered on summits of active p63-bound (co-occupied by p63 and H3K27ac) regions. (B) ChIP-seq tracks showing the co-localization of BRDT and p63 at FAT2, KRT14 and PTHLH loci. (C) CoIP showing BRDT interacts with p63. (D) Venn diagrams showing the overlap between BRDT- and p63-targets in KYSE180 (left) and TE6 (right). (E) Quantitative real-time PCR analysis of FAT2, KRT14 and PTHLH upon knock-down of p63 in KYSE180. GAPDH was used to normalize gene expression. Data are represented as mean ± SD, n=3. Unpaired t-test was used. (F) Quantification of migrated cells upon knock-down of p63 and FAT2 in KYSE180. Data are represented as mean ± SD, n=2. Unpaired one-way ANOVA test followed by Dunnett's test was used. ****: P≤0.0001, ***: P≤0.005, **: P≤0.01, *: P≤0.05, ns: not significant.

2.3.5 BRDT directs and rewires ΔNp63-dependent transcription in ESCC

The expression of ΔNp63 is a common feature among squamous cell carcinomas, including ESCC. Thus, we were interested in determining the specificity of BRDT in controlling ΔNp63-dependent transcription and the impact of BRDT on the ΔNp63-dependent program. Therefore, we depleted ΔNp63 in KYSE150 ESCC cells, which lack endogenous BRDT expression, and compared this dataset with genes down-regulated following BRDT and ΔNp63 depletion in KYSE180 cells. Strikingly, we found that BRDT/ΔNp63 dependent genes displayed limited overlap with ΔNp63 targets from KYSE150 cells (Fig. 20A), indicating that BRDT may function to reprogram ΔNp63 dependencies in ESCC. We further compared the expression level of BRDT/ΔNp63 targets and found that these genes are more highly expressed in KYSE180 compared with KYSE150 and were not regulated by ΔNp63 in KYSE150 (Fig. 20B), further supporting that BRDT specifically reprograms the ΔNp63-dependent transcriptional program. To further investigate the ability of BRDT to reprogram ΔNp63 dependencies, we performed RNA-seq in KYSE150 cells over-expressing BRDT. In accordance with our hypothesis, a subset of BRDT/ΔNp63 targets were up-regulated upon over-expression of BRDT in KYSE150 cells (Fig. 20C). Consistently, many BRDT/ΔNp63 target genes were enriched in cells over-expressing BRDT, suggesting that over-expressing BRDT in a BRDT-negative cell line is sufficient to partially reprogram the ΔNp63-dependent transcriptional program (Fig. 20D). To further confirm the importance of ΔNp63 in directing the BRDT function in ESCC, we depleted ΔNp63 in either control KYSE150 cells or cells overexpressing BRDT, and examined ΔNp63/BRDT target gene expression. Consistent with our model in which ΔNp63 sequence-specifically directs BRDT to target genes, we observed that depletion of ΔNp63 precludes the ability of BRDT to activate the expression of either *KRT14* or *FAT2* (Fig. 20E). Importantly, consistent with a functional importance of BRDT in controlling tumor cell migration, BRDT overexpression in KYSE150 increased cell migration (Fig. 20F, Additional file 1: Fig. S3). Collectively, we showed that BRDT rewires the ΔNp63-dependent transcription programs in ESCC.

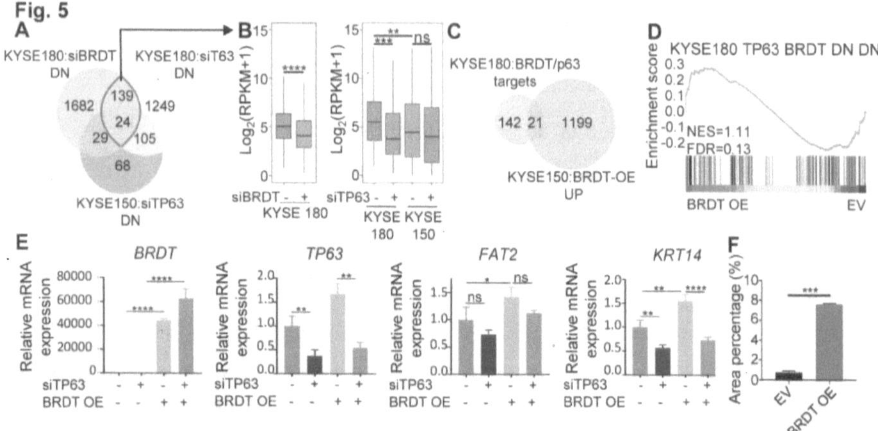

Fig. 5 BRDT directs and rewires ΔNp63 programs. (A) Venn diagram showing the overlap between the BRDT/p63-targets in KYSE180 and p63-targets in KYSE150. Red circle denotes BRDT/p63-targets. (B) Boxplots showing the expression of BRDT/p63-targets in different conditions in KYSE180 and KYSE150. Paired t-test was used for the left panel and paired one-way ANOVA test followed by Tukey's test was used for right panel. (C) Venn diagram showing the overlap between the BRDT/p63-targets of KYSE180 and BRDT-activated genes of KYSE150. (D) GSEA showing that BRDT/p63-targets are enriched in KYSE150 over-expressing BRDT. EV: empty vector. (E) Quantitative real-time PCR analysis of FAT2 and KRT14 upon over-expression of BRDT and knock–down of p63 in KYSE150. GAPDH was used to normalize gene expression. Data are represented as mean ± SD, n=3. Unpaired one-way ANOVA test followed by Tukey's test was used. (F) Quantification of migrated cells upon over-expression of BRDT in KYSE150. Data are represented as mean ± SD, n=2. Unpaired t-test was used. ****: P≤0.0001, ***: P≤0.005, **: P≤0.01, *: P≤0.05, ns: not significant.

2.3.6 BRDT controls ΔNp63-dependent super enhancers

We and others previously demonstrated that ΔNp63 plays a central role in determining tumor cell identity by controlling large genomic regions highly enriched for the occupancy of the BET protein BRD4 referred to as super enhancers, to modulate target gene expression (Hamdan and Johnsen, 2018; Hnisz et al., 2014; Jiang et al., 2018; Lovén et al., 2013). Given our findings that BRDT co-localized with ΔNp63 on several genes such as *FAT2* and *PTHLH*, which we previously demonstrated as being associated with ΔNp63-dependent super enhancers in pancreatic cancer (Hamdan and Johnsen, 2018), we investigated whether BRDT, like BRD4, may be a defining feature of super enhancers in a subset of ESCC. For this, we used the gold standard ROSE algorithm to compare the ability of BRD4, BRDT or ΔNp63 occupancy to identify super enhancers on stitched H3K27ac peaks (Lovén et al., 2013; Whyte et al., 2013) (Fig. 21A). Strikingly, we found that more than 60% of the BRDT-occupied super enhancers overlap with those identified by either BRD4 or ΔNp63 occupancy (Fig. 21B).

Recent studies have revealed that super enhancers direct specific transcriptional programs via chromatin loops with the promoters of important target genes (Beagrie et al., 2017; Lovén et al., 2013; Schmitt et al., 2016). In order to accurately identify genes associated with BRDT super enhancers, we utilized HiChIP (Mumbach et al., 2016) to capture chromatin interactions associated with active (H3K27ac occupied) chromatin regions in KYSE180. Interestingly, the identified BRDT super enhancers are associated with key BRDT/ΔNp63-dependent subtype-specific and migration-associated genes such as *FAT2*, *KRT14* and *PTHLH* (Fig. 21C). Moreover, we exploited HiChIP data to identify genes associated with super enhancers and found these genes to be enriched in control KYSE180 cells compared to the BRDT-depleted group (Fig. 21D), highlighting the role of BRDT in directing super enhancer function.

BET proteins have provided an important paradigm as therapeutic epigenetic targets in cancer (Lovén et al., 2013). Thus, given its amenability to BET inhibitor treatment (Gaucher et al., 2012; Matzuk et al., 2012), BRDT may therefore represent a very attractive target for precision medicine in ESCC. In particular, proteolysis targeting chimeric (PROTAC) molecules represent novel candidates for anti-cancer therapy (Winter et al., 2015). Notably, the VHL-dependent PROTAC MZ1 was reported to display specificity towards BRD4 in comparison to BRD2 and BRD3 (Zengerle et al., 2015). However, to what degree it affects BRDT is currently unknown. Interestingly, our results demonstrate that MZ1 rapidly and potently promotes the selective degradation of BRDT. We found that BRDT was completely degraded after a brief treatment with 1 µM MZ1, while BRD4 expression was greatly, but not completely decreased, and BRD2 and BRD3 protein levels were comparatively unaffected (Fig. 21E). Based on these findings we tested whether MZ1 treatment can also downregulate the expression of BRDT/ΔNp63 targets. In order to test this, we examined the expression of nascent (heterogeneous nuclear) RNA (hnRNA) of three BRDT/ΔNp63 target genes (*KRT14*, *FAT2* and *PTHLH*) following MZ1 treatment (Fig. 21F). Indeed, these results resemble the effects observed following the knock-down of BRDT or ΔNp63. Together, these results show that BRDT occupies a subset of ΔNp63-dependent SEs to modulate squamous-specific gene expression in a subset of ESCC.

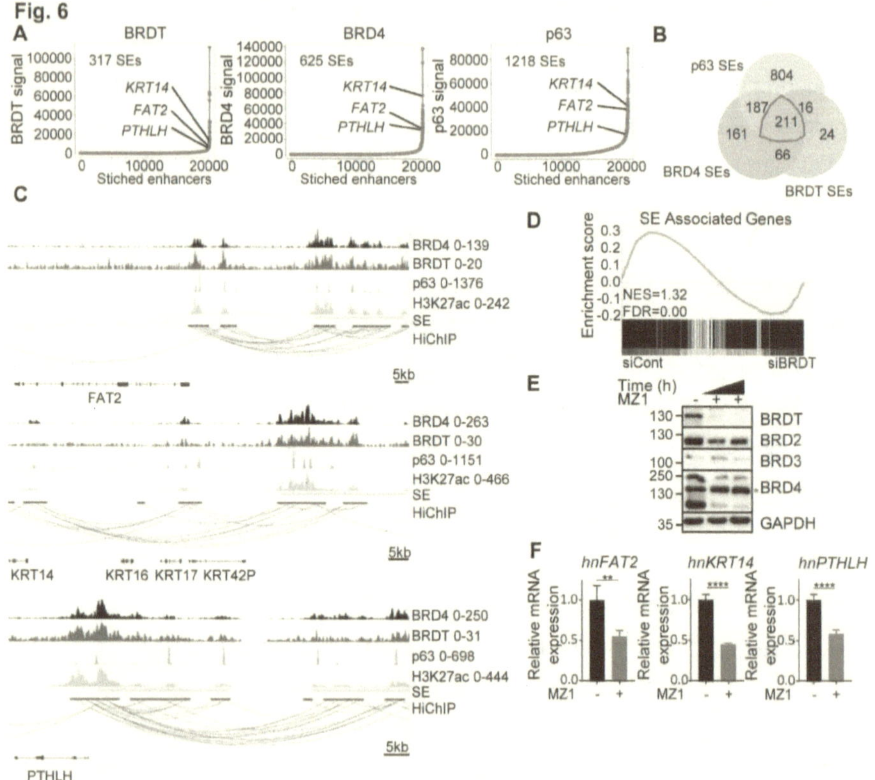

Fig. 6 BRDT controls ΔNp63-dependent super enhancers. (A) Super enhancer calling using BRDT, BRD4 and p63, respectively. (B) Venn diagram showing the overlap among BRDT-, BRD4- and p63- super enhancers. (C) Tracks showing BRDT, BRD4, p63, H3K27ac, super enhancers (SE) and H3K27ac HiChIP interactions at *FAT2*, *KRT14* and *PTHLH* loci. (D) GSEA showing genes associated with super enhancers are enriched in control group in KYSE180. (E) Western blot analysis of BET proteins upon 4h and 8h of 1 μM MZ1 treatment in KYSE180. *: non-specific band. (F) Quantitative real-time PCR analysis of heterogeneous nuclear RNA of *FAT2*, *KRT14* and *PTHLH* upon 8h of 1 μM MZ1 treatment in KYSE180. *GAPDH* was used to normalize gene expression. Data are represented as mean ± SD, n=4. Unpaired t-test was used. ****: $P \leq 0.0001$, ***: $P \leq 0.005$, **: $P \leq 0.01$, *: $P \leq 0.05$, ns: not significant.

2.4 DISCUSSION

Current therapeutic approaches for the treatment of ESCC display highly heterogeneous efficacies and frequently elicit numerous undesirable side effects. The identification of therapeutic targets with high tissue specificity would afford a unique opportunity to cancer therapy with low-toxicity and decreased side effects. In this work, we sought to ascertain such targets by identifying variably expressed tissue-specific epigenetic factors aberrantly expressed in ESCC. Utilizing an unbiased approach, we identified *BRDT*, the testis-specific member of BET proteins, as one of the most variably expressed tissue-specific genes in ESCC. While depletion of BRDT did not impair cell proliferation, it did result in attenuated cell migration and downregulation of related pathways. Mechanistically, we demonstrate for the first time that BRDT occupancy is associated with the activity of a select set of cancer subtype-specific genes. Integrative analyses of the transcriptomic and genomic occupancy data led us to the finding that BRDT acts at a subset of super enhancers to maintain the expression of cell lineage-specific genes.

BRDT has been reported to function as a master regulator during spermatogenesis by inducing massive chromatin reorganization (Pivot-Pajot et al., 2003). Interestingly, BRDT was also reported to be ectopically expressed in cancer two decades ago (Scanlan et al., 2000), but its function in tumorigenesis has remained elusive until now. We show for the first time that BRDT can regulate transcription by promoting ΔNp63 function at certain super enhancers. This regulatory mechanism is similar to what we have previously shown for BRD4, the closest paralog to BRDT, which localizes to lineage-specific enhancers to regulate genes which are crucial for lineage specification (Najafova et al., 2017) and pancreatic cancer subtype (Hamdan and Johnsen, 2018). Consistently, we report that BRDT localizes to a select subset of ΔNp63-bound super enhancers, serving to maintain the expression of some squamous-specific genes. While the precise function of BRDT at enhancers remains to be determined, like BRD4, BRDT possesses an extended carboxyl terminus that can interact with positive-transcriptional elongation factor-b (P-TEFb) (Gaucher et al., 2012). Thus, it is likely that BRDT may function to control enhancer activity via regulation of promoter proximal pausing and/or enhancer RNA synthesis, both of which are primarily controlled by the P-TEFb subunit CDK9 in conjunction with BET proteins (Kanno et al., 2014; Moon et al., 2005).

A number of studies have reported an anti-tumor activity of BET inhibition in preclinical models (Aird et al., 2017; Cheng et al., 2013; Filippakopoulos et al., 2010; Segura et al., 2013), thus leading to numerous ongoing early phase clinical trials of BET inhibitors in various cancers. A phase I clinical study has already shown that BET inhibitors can bring clinical benefits in different cancer entities including NUT midline carcinoma, colorectal cancer and prostate cancer (Piha-Paul et al., 2020). This highlights the potential of developing BET inhibition as a novel therapeutic approach for cancer treatment. However, BET inhibitors elicit a number of side effects related to their physiological roles in hematopoietic cell lineage specification (Bolden et al., 2014). Recently, new inhibitors developed specifically against the second bromodomain of BRD4 show a much lower toxicity, but also a more limited spectrum of malignant indications (Faivre et al., 2020; Gilan et al., 2020). Nevertheless, these studies provide a precedent for the feasibility of developing specific inhibitors for the individual bromodomains of BET proteins, therefore suggesting a specific targeting of BRDT may be possible. Another potential therapeutic approach is through the utilization of BET isoform-specific PROTACs. In general, BET degraders confer a more profound effect on BET-mediated transcriptional modulation, thus leading to a stronger antitumor activity (Bai et al., 2017; Raina et al., 2016). One notable example is MZ1, a PROTAC BET degrader which was previously shown to preferentially degrade BRD4 over BRD2 and BRD3 (Zengerle et al., 2015). Interestingly, our results demonstrate that MZ1 efficiently induces BRDT degradation to an extent even greater than BRD4 and efficiently downregulates BRDT-dependent transcriptional targets. Thus, specific inhibition or degradation of BRDT represents a unique opportunity with a strong potential for clinical application in a subset of ESCC.

In our study BRDT was specifically required for cell migration, but appeared to be dispensable for cell proliferation. Therefore, despite the potential utility of small molecule inhibitors or PROTACs in blocking BET protein function, it is currently unclear whether the inhibition or depletion of BRDT activity would be sufficient to impede ESCC tumor growth. Thus, while such inhibitors would be predicted to limit tumor metastasis, a different approach would likely be required to more efficiently impede tumor growth. One potential approach may be the conjugation of anti-neoplastic substances such as chemotherapeutic agents or radionuclides to a BRDT-specific ligand. Such an approach would not only enable highly specific targeting of BRDT-expressing tumor cells, but could also facilitate non-invasive imaging of tumors as well. Similar proof of principle molecules have been developed for hormone-dependent cancers such as breast and prostate cancer by utilizing specific conjugates of estrogen and androgen receptor ligands, respectively (Han et al., 2014; Vultos et al., 2017). Importantly, given the unique tissue specificity of BRDT expression during spermatogenesis, it is anticipated that any side effects due to its specific targeting will both be minimal and reversible.

2.5 CONCLUSIONS

Taken together, our unbiased screening of epigenetic factors led us to the identification of a testis-specific BET protein, BRDT, as an unexpected and novel potential therapeutic target in ESCC. Future studies will be needed to identify and refine small molecule probes targeting BRDT and test their utility in pre-clinical models and early clinical trials.

2.6 METHODS

2.6.1 Cell culture

Cells were cultured in a humidified incubator supplied with 5% CO_2 at 37°C. RPMI-1640 (Invitrogen) with 10% FBS (Sigma) and 1% penicillin/streptomycin (Sigma) was used to culture KYSE70, KYSE180 and TE6 cells. RPMI/F12 medium (Invitrogen) with 5% FBS (Sigma) and 1% penicillin/streptomycin (Sigma) was used to culture KYSE150 cells. Knock-down, knock-out, over-expression and proliferation assay are described in Additional file 1: Supplemental Methods.

2.6.2 Migration assay

Cell culture inserts with 8µm transparent PET membrane (Corning, Inc) were pre-equilibrated in serum-free medium for 30 minutes prior to being placed in 24-well companion plates (Corining, Inc). 1 ml of normal medium was placed in the well and 50,000 cells in 500 µL were seeded in the inserts and incubated for 48 hours. The migrated cells were then stained with 1% crystal violet in 20% ethanol for 15 minutes after removing remaining non-migrated cells from the inner side of inserts and fixing with methanol for 20 min. Subsequently, inserts were dried, scanned and quantified with ImageJ.

2.6.3 Tissue specificity expression analysis

The tissue specificity is evaluated according to the published work (Wells et al., 2015) with minor modifications. The maximal p-value of specificity index (pSI) across all tissues was taken to calculate tissue specificity index (TSI). The formula is as following: $TSI = -\log_{10}(\max(pSI))$.

2.6.4 Patient samples, RNA isolation, quantitative real-time PCR (qPCR), RNA-seq library preparation

31 pairs of fresh tumor and adjacent non-tumor samples of ESCC patients prior to treatment were collected and subject to snap freezing at Osaka University Hospital, Osaka, Japan. RNA was isolated using QIAzol regents (Qiagen). RNA-seq library preparation was performed using TruSeq RNA library prep kit V2 (Illumina). Briefly, after verification of the RNA quality with electrophoresis, 500 ng of RNA was used as starting material to prepare RNA-seq libraries using TruSeq RNA library prep kit V2 (Illumina) following the manufacturer's manual. RNA-seq libraries were quantified using Qubit 2 (Invitrogen) and were subjected to Bioanalyzer 2100 (Agilent) for fragment analysis. The sequencing was done by NGS Integrative Genomics Core Unit (NIG) in Göttingen, Germany and Genome Analysis Core in Rochester, Minnesota, USA. More details are provided in Additional file 1: Supplemental Methods.

2.6.5 RNA-seq analysis

Sequencing reads obtained from sequencing facilities were first subjected to FASTQC (available at https://www.bioinformatics.babraham.ac.uk/projects/fastqc/) for quality control. Reads were then mapped to human genome (hg38) with STAR (Dobin et al., 2013). After sorting the BAM files using samtools (Li et al., 2009a), the feature counting was done by HTSeq (Anders et al., 2015). The resulting count files were used for differential gene expression analysis with DESeq2 package (Love et al., 2014). Gene set enrichment analysis (GSEA) was conducted using GSEA program (Subramanian et al., 2005). EnrichR (Chen et al., 2013) was used to analyze enriched pathways and transcription factors.

2.6.6 Co-immunoprecipitation (CoIP)

Cells were treated with 20 nM bortezomib for 12 hours prior to harvest using co-IP buffer (50 mM Tris-HCl, 1% NP-40, 150 mM NaCl) with the same protease inhibitors used in ChIP. Cells were then lysed for 10 minutes on ice and scraped. The cell lysate was sonicated for three cycles of 5 minutes using a Biorupter (Diagenode). The sonicated lysate was then centrifuged to collect supernatant which was further split for immunoprecipitation. The pre-clearing process was performed by incubating samples with 60 µL of sepharose beads (50%) at 4°C for 1 hour on a rotator. The samples were then centrifuged mildly to collect supernatant. Antibodies were then added to the supernatant and the mix was rotated on at 4°C overnight. The quantity of antibody used in this study was provided in Additional file 6: Table S5. 50 µL of protein G-coupled sepharose beads (50%) (GE healthcare) was then added to samples and the samples were then incubated at 4°C for 2 hours to pull down the immune complex. Subsequently, samples were centrifuged and washed three times with co-IP buffer. Finally, the collected beads were eluted by adding 25 µL of laemmli buffer and subjected to western blot for analyzing protein interactions.

2.6.7 Chromatin immunoprecipitation (ChIP) and ChIP-seq library preparation

ChIP was done as previously described (Hamdan and Johnsen, 2018; Najafova et al., 2017) with minor changes. In brief, cells were washed with PBS and cross-linked using 1% formaldehyde in PBS for 10 minutes. After quenching the formaldehyde with 1.25mM glycine, fixed cells were washed twice with ice-cold PBS. Cells were then lysed using nuclear preparation buffer supplied with protease inhibitors to harvest nuclei. After brief centrifugation, the nuclear preparation was replaced by lysis buffer containing protease inhibitors. Subsequently, samples were sonicated for 12 cycles using Biorupter (Diagenode). The supernatant was taken after a short centrifugation for a pre-clearing process, in which sepharose 4B (GE Healthcare) beads were co-incubated for 1 hour. The antibody was then added to the pre-cleared chromatin for overnight incubation. The information of antibodies used in this study is provided in Additional file 6: table S5. Sepharose beads coupled with Protein A or Protein G (GE Healthcare) were then added to the reaction and incubated for 2 hours to pull down the immunocomplex. The samples were then washed with lysis buffer, wash buffer and TE buffer. De-crosslinking was done by incubating with 20 µg proteinase K overnight. The DNA was extracted using phenol/choloroform/isoamyl alcohol (25:24:1) and precipitated using ethanol.

ChIP-seq library preparation was done using KAPA Hyper Prep Kit (Roche). ChIP DNA was quantified with Qubit (Invitrogen). The ChIP-seq library preparation was prepared using the KAPA Hyper Prep Kit (Roche) and following manufacturer's instruction. The library concentration and fragment size were determined by Qubit and Bioanalyzer, respectively. The sequencing was done by NGS Integrative Genomics Core Unit (NIG) in Göttingen, Germany.

2.6.8 ChIP-seq bioinformatic analysis

The sequencing reads were mapped to human genome (hg19) using bowtie (Langmead et al., 2009). The resulting bam files were sorted and indexed using samtools (Li et al., 2009a). Deeptools (Ramírez et al., 2014) were used to convert bam files to signal tracks. The bigwig file of BRDT was smoothened by averaging five consecutive bins. MACS2 (Zhang et al., 2008) was utilized to identify peaks and motif analysis was run using the homer program suit (Heinz et al., 2010). Notably, BRDT peaks were called using the following parameters: --broad --broad-cutoff 0.1 --llocal 50000 due to low sigal/background ratio. The identification of super enhancers was carried out by ROSE (Lovén et al., 2013; Whyte et al., 2013). ChromHMM (Ernst and Kellis, 2012) was used to analyze the histone marking pattern of genome.

2.6.9 H3K27ac HiChIP

HiChIP was done as previously described (Mumbach et al., 2016) with some changes. Cells were washed twice with PBS and cross-linked using 1% formaldehyde in PBS for 10 minutes, which was quenched by incubating with 1.25 mM glycine solution for 5 minutes. The cross-linked cells were washed twice with ice-cold PBS and lysed with Hi-C lysis buffer. The nuclei were collected and resuspended in 0.5% SDS, which was then quenched by adding 10% Triton X-100. The digestion was carried out by incubating with 200U of MboI, DpnII and HinfI (NEB) at 37°C for 2 hours. After heat inactivating the restriction enzymes at 62°C for 10 min, the overhangs of digested chromatin were filled by adding dCTP, dGTP, dTTP and biotin labeled dATP (Jena biosciences) and DNA polymerase I Large (Klenow) Fragment (NEB). After the biotin incorporation, proximity ligation was performed using T4 DNA Ligase (NEB). The samples were then resuspended in lysis buffer supplemented with protease inhibitors. To better solubilize the chromatin, 4 cycles of sonication were applied. The size distribution of DNA fragments was verified with electrophoresis before pre-clearing the chromatin with 50% sepharose 4B (GE Healthcare) slurry in lysis buffer. H3K27ac-associated chromatin was captured by adding 6 µg of H3K27ac antibody (Diagenode). Protein A-sepharose (GE Healthcare) beads were added to capture the immunocomplex. The beads were subsequently washed with lysis buffer, wash buffer, lysis buffer and TE buffer and subjected to DNA extraction with phenol/chloroform/isoamyl alcohol (25:24:1) as previously described in the section of ChIP. Right-sided size selection using KAPApure beads (Roche) was utilized according to manufacturer's guidelines to exclude big DNA fragments prior to library preparation. The right-sided size selected DNA was then used for library preparation following the KAPA Hyper Prep manual. Streptavidin T-1 beads (Invitrogen) was washed with Tween Wash Buffer and resuspended in Biotin Binding Buffer to capture biotin-labeled DNA. Library amplification was carried out according to the KAPA Hyper Prep manual. The fragment distribution of HiChIP libraries was determined using Bioanalyzer (Agilent). The libraries were then sequenced by Genome Analysis Core at Mayo Clinic, MN, USA.

2.6.10 HiChIP bioinformatic analysis

The HiChIP data was analyzed using the HiC-Pro pipeline (Servant et al., 2015) which includes read alignment, HiC read filtering, quality checks and contact matrix building. FitHiChIP (Bhattacharyya et al., 2019) was utilized to identify active p63-associated loops. The "Peak-To-All" mode was used and the resulting loops were further processed to exclude those of which either end is not marked by H3K27ac. Subsequently, the result was converted to bedpe format for downstream visualization and enhancer-gene association. The enhancer-gene association was done using in-house scripts and the link to the source code can be found in the section of "Availability of data and materials".

2.6.11 Statistical analyses

Data are presented as mean ± SD. Statistical methods, number of replicates and significance were indicated in each experiment.

2.7 ABBREVIATIONS

ESCC: Esophageal squamous cell carcinoma; EAC: Esophageal adenocarcinoma; BET: Bromodomain and Extraterminal; BRDT: Bromodomain Testis-specific protein; SE: Super enhancer; CCLE: Cancer Cell Line Encyclopedia; ECM: Extracellular matrix; GSEA: Gene set enrichment analysis; CoIP: Co-immunoprecipitation; ChIP: Chromatin Immunoprecipitation; HiChIP: Hi-C followed by chromatin immunoprecipitation; hnRNA: heterogeneous nuclear RNA; PROTAC: Proteolysis-targeting chimera; P-TEFb: Positive-transcriptional elongation factor-b

2.8 DECLARATIONS

2.8.1 Ethics approval and consent to participate

This study was approved by the appropriate institutional review boards of Osaka University Hospital (approval number: O8226-10).

2.8.2 Availability of data and materials

An in-house script for associating genes with super enhancers is available in the GitHub repository CCLE data can be found at The data discussed in this publication have been deposited in NCBI's Gene Expression Omnibus (Edgar et al., 2002) and are accessible through GEO Series accession number GSE155187.

2.8.3 Competing interests

Not applicable.

2.8.4 Funding

This work was supported by the *Gertrud and Erich Roggenbuck Foundation* (to S.A.J.). X.W. was supported by the *China Scholarship Council* (201606300011 to X.W.) and the *International Max Planck Research School for Genome Science* (travel expenses to X.W.).

2.8.5 Authors' contributions

S.A.J. and X.W. designed research; X.W., A.P.K., M.Y., E.P., P.B., F.H.H. performed research; X.W. analyzed data; K.T. and Y.K. contributed reagents and materials; X.W. and S.A.J. wrote the manuscript. All authors read and approved the final manuscript.

2.9 ADDITIONAL FILES

2.9.1 Additional file 1: Supplemental Figures (Fig. S1-3) and Supplemental Methods.

2.9.1.1 Supplemental Figures

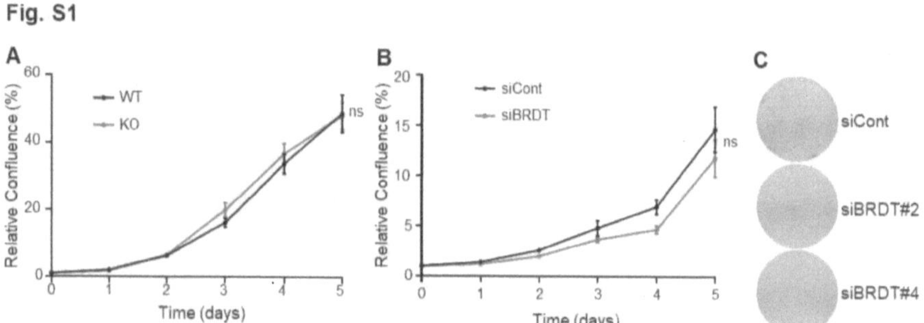

Fig. S1 Growth kinetics analysis of CRISPR/Cas9-mediated knock-out of BRDT in KYSE180 (A) and siRNA-mediated knock-down of BRDT in TE6 (B). Data are represented as mean ± SD, n=5. Paired t-test was used. ****: $P \leq 0.0001$, ***: $P \leq 0.005$, **: $P \leq 0.01$, *: $P \leq 0.05$, ns: not significant. (C) Representative staining of migrated cells upon BRDT knock-down with different siRNAs in KYSE180.

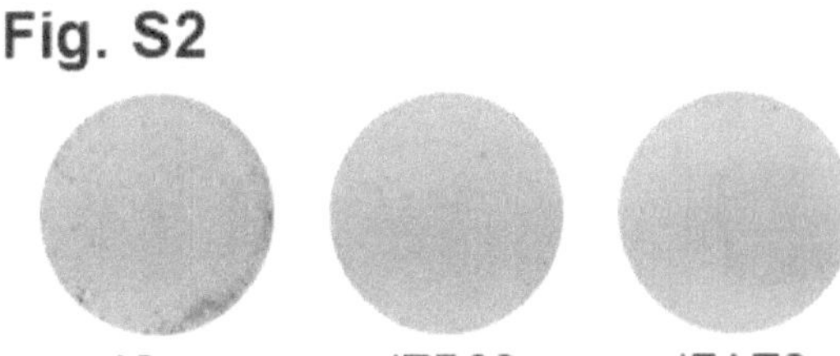

Fig. S2 Representative images of migrated cells upon knock-down of p63 and FAT2 in KYSE180.

Fig. S3

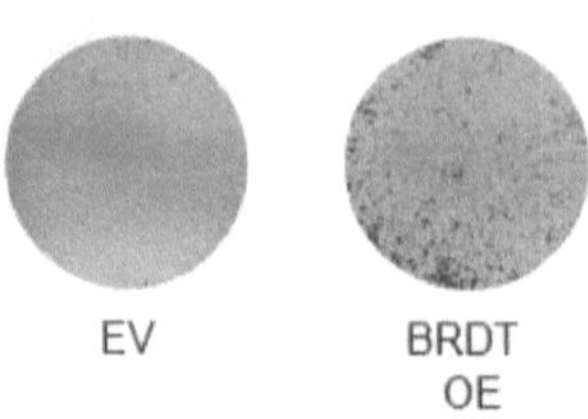

Fig. S3 Representative images of migrated cells upon over-expression of BRDT in KYSE150.

2.9.1.2 Supplemental Methods

2.9.1.2.1 Cell culture, knock-down, knock-out and over-expression

KYSE70, KYSE150 and KYSE180 cells were provided by Jessica Eggert (University Medical Center Göttingen, Germany). TE6 cells were provided by Dr. Koji Tanaka (Osaka University, Japan). Cells were cultured in a humidified incubator supplied with 5% CO_2 at 37°C. RPMI-1640 (Invitrogen) with 10% FBS (Sigma) and 1% penicillin/streptomycin (Sigma) was used to culture KYSE70, KYSE180 and TE6 cells. RPMI/F12 medium (Invitrogen) with 5% FBS (Sigma) and 1% penicillin/streptomycin (Sigma) was used to culture KYSE150 cells. siRNA-mediated knock-down was performed using Lipofectamine RNAiMAX (Invitrogen) and following manufacturer's instructions. The sequence information of siGENOME siRNAs (Dharmacon) employed is provided in Additional file 4: table S3. CRISPR/Cas9 mediated knock-out was carried out as previously described (Sen et al., 2019) and the gRNA information is provided in Additional file 3: table S2. The over-expression experiments for RNA-seq were performed by electroporation as previously described (Sen et al., 2019). The simultaneous over-expression of BRDT and knock-down of ΔNp63 was carried out using Lipofectamine 3000 (Invitrogen) according to manufacturer's instructions. The control vector pCDNA5/TO was a gift from Prof. Matthias Dobbelstein (University Medical Center Göttingen, Germany) and the BRDT over-expression plasmid was a gift from Kyle Miller (Addgene plasmid # 65381 ; ; RRID:Addgene_65381) (Gong et al., 2015).

2.9.1.2.2 Proliferation assay

1,000 cells were seeded in 96-well plates (Corning) and incubated for 5 to 7 days. Cells were imaged and their confluence assessed every 24 hours by Celigo (Brooks Life Sciences System, USA). Each measuring point was normalized to the corresponding confluence measurement at day 0.

2.9.1.2.3 RNA isolation and quantitative real-time PCR (qPCR)

Patient materials were homogenized using Tissue Lyser (Qiagen). QIAzol was added to cells or lysed tissue, which once lysed were transferred to a new tube. Chloroform (1/5 volume of QIAzol reagent) was added to the tube and the mixture was vortexed thoroughly. After centrifugation, the aqueous phase was transferred to a new tube and an equal volume of isopropanol was added to precipitate RNA. The RNA pellet was washed with 70% ethanol in DEPC water and resuspended in DEPC water. The concentration of RNA was measured using Nanodrop (Denovox). 1µg RNA was used for reverse transcription with M-MuLV reverse transcriptase (NEB) and 1.5 µM 9-mer random primers. For reverse transcription of patient RNA, Reverse Transcription System (Promega) was used. The complementary DNA (cDNA) was then subjected to the following PCR program: 95°C for 2 minutes, 40 cycles of 10 seconds at 95 °C followed by 30 seconds at 60 °C to determine gene expression. *GAPDH* and *ACTB* were used for normalizing qPCR results in Göttingen and Osaka, respectively. The melting curve was determined by reading plates every 0.5 °C from 60 °C to 95 °C. Primers for qPCR experiments were designed with NCBI Primer BLAST (Ye et al., 2012). The primer sequences are listed in Additional file 5: table S4.

2.9.1.2.4 Protein isolation and western blot

Protein was isolated by adding RIPA buffer (1% NP40, 0.1% SDS, 0.5 sodium deoxycholate in 1 x PBS) containing protease inhibitors (100 µM N-Ethylmaleimeide, 100 µM Pefabloc, 100 µM β-glycerophosphate and 1 µM Aprotinin/Leupeptin). The protein samples were subjected to sonication (Bioruptor Pico, Diagenode) at high frequency for 10 minutes (30 seconds on and 30 seconds off). The protein was mixed with 6x Lämmli buffer (350 mM Tris-HCl, 30% glycerol, 10% SDS, 9.3% DTT and 0.02% bromophenol blue) and the mixture was heated at 95°C for 5 minutes. The protein samples were then loaded to a polyacrylamide gel and run for separation. After transferring the protein to nitrocellulose membranes (GE Healthcare), the membrane was blocked with 5% milk in 1x TBST (20 mM Tris, 14 mM NaCl, 0.1% Tween 20) prior to overnight incubation with primary antibodes listed in Additional file 6: Table S5. The respective secondary antibody was incubated with the membrane for 1 hour prior to imaging using BioRad gel doc (Biorad).

2.9.2 Additional file 2: Table S1: Variance of expression and tissue specificity index of epigenetic factors.

Gene ID	Gene name	pSI (Max)	TSI	Variance (TCGA ESCC)
ENSG00000148584	A1CF	0.014348	1.843213896	0.023180499
ENSG00000136518	ACTL6A	0.984172	0.006929092	0.346097459

ENSG00000077080	ACTL6B	0.063658	1.196145844	0.045402158
ENSG00000133627	ACTR3B	0.963233	0.01626861	0.206689644
ENSG00000101442	ACTR5	0.917232	0.037520932	0.165924474
ENSG00000075089	ACTR6	0.986767	0.005785576	0.177365146
ENSG00000113812	ACTR8	0.833754	0.078962198	0.086791249
ENSG00000101126	ADNP	0.82664	0.082683385	0.132219654
ENSG00000139154	AEBP2	0.943549	0.025235589	0.250457528
ENSG00000111732	AICDA	3.02E-05	4.520483533	0.084179717
ENSG00000160224	AIRE	0.113623	0.944533028	0.229794356
ENSG00000100601	ALKBH1	0.908221	0.041808528	0.097573827
ENSG00000140350	ANP32A	0.994609	0.002347748	0.165863477
ENSG00000136938	ANP32B	0.946841	0.023723137	0.250011319
ENSG00000143401	ANP32E	0.993116	0.003000047	0.271554866
ENSG00000166313	APBB1	0.999905	4.11673E-05	0.713907438
ENSG00000100823	APEX1	0.995188	0.002094692	0.254414059
ENSG00000111701	APOBEC1	3E-05	4.523095838	0.032645226
ENSG00000124701	APOBEC2	0.937143	0.028194201	0.040711967
ENSG00000128383	APOBEC3A	0.925699	0.033530164	2.514286713
ENSG00000179750	APOBEC3B	0.89368	0.048817844	0.995273207
ENSG00000244509	APOBEC3C	0.996304	0.001608265	0.3128847
ENSG00000243811	APOBEC3D	0.992914	0.003088317	0.403887054
ENSG00000128394	APOBEC3F	0.992515	0.003262773	0.366432456
ENSG00000239713	APOBEC3G	0.999746	0.000110136	0.854383345
ENSG00000100298	APOBEC3H	0.890486	0.050372747	0.110510682
ENSG00000117713	ARID1A	0.835966	0.077811252	0.174934293
ENSG00000049618	ARID1B	0.966493	0.014801398	0.119159756
ENSG00000189079	ARID2	0.919417	0.036487386	0.197384691
ENSG00000116017	ARID3A	0.961581	0.017014331	0.375744043
ENSG00000032219	ARID4A	0.934522	0.029410591	0.264682153
ENSG00000054267	ARID4B	0.904432	0.043623913	0.213378104
ENSG00000196843	ARID5A	0.984692	0.006699455	0.459174346
ENSG00000150347	ARID5B	0.991727	0.003607931	0.460837056
ENSG00000133794	ARNTL	0.932006	0.030581276	0.208988676
ENSG00000137486	ARRB1	0.99629	0.001614292	0.49283622
ENSG00000111875	ASF1A	0.850908	0.070117538	0.332431209
ENSG00000105011	ASF1B	0.962674	0.016520886	0.502187903
ENSG00000116539	ASH1L	0.923096	0.034752958	0.224913574
ENSG00000129691	ASH2L	0.933895	0.029702072	0.408606944
ENSG00000171456	ASXL1	0.962347	0.016668472	0.191297181
ENSG00000143970	ASXL2	0.914757	0.038694335	0.344767651
ENSG00000141431	ASXL3	0.849626	0.070772334	0.082486558
ENSG00000156802	ATAD2	0.932309	0.030440195	0.427666054
ENSG00000119778	ATAD2B	0.948236	0.023083471	0.156519887
ENSG00000171681	ATF7IP	0.877391	0.056806674	0.243043176

ENSG00000149311	ATM	0.946244	0.023996835	0.356070159
ENSG00000111676	ATN1	0.984754	0.006672413	0.278692295
ENSG00000175054	ATR	0.902697	0.044457923	0.338897306
ENSG00000163635	ATXN7	0.948037	0.0231748	0.168910017
ENSG00000087152	ATXN7L3	0.866391	0.062286079	0.149747301
ENSG00000087586	AURKA	0.962727	0.016496725	0.290791232
ENSG00000178999	AURKB	0.93219	0.030495405	0.446899974
ENSG00000105146	AURKC	0.951922	0.021398672	0.096930465
ENSG00000105393	BABAM1	0.908939	0.041465074	0.155709219
ENSG00000140320	BAHD1	0.939937	0.026901297	0.140961021
ENSG00000172530	BANP	0.821554	0.085363967	0.086274534
ENSG00000163930	BAP1	0.893213	0.049044861	0.203992932
ENSG00000138376	BARD1	0.985108	0.00651629	0.219227838
ENSG00000198604	BAZ1A	0.997515	0.001080418	0.373078652
ENSG00000009954	BAZ1B	0.898457	0.04650276	0.187329418
ENSG00000076108	BAZ2A	0.957132	0.019028208	0.166658021
ENSG00000123636	BAZ2B	0.869494	0.060733175	0.33264886
ENSG00000168283	BMI1	0.994274	0.002493721	0.206757393
ENSG00000171634	BPTF	0.908657	0.041599934	0.165752512
ENSG00000012048	BRCA1	0.920623	0.035918132	0.381383533
ENSG00000139618	BRCA2	0.830121	0.08085868	0.3716988
ENSG00000100425	BRD1	0.899985	0.045764914	0.196755825
ENSG00000204256	BRD2	0.876516	0.057239988	0.10229468
ENSG00000169925	BRD3	0.791483	0.101558601	0.217615962
ENSG00000141867	BRD4	0.913604	0.039241868	0.181003965
ENSG00000166164	BRD7	0.898515	0.046474664	0.092962933
ENSG00000112983	BRD8	0.897489	0.046971033	0.146295233
ENSG00000028310	BRD9	0.8114	0.090764997	0.301200031
ENSG00000137948	BRDT	2.9E-05	4.537819095	1.285502064
ENSG00000158019	BRE	0.890737	0.050250584	0.147065069
ENSG00000174744	BRMS1	0.907462	0.042171549	0.345814648
ENSG00000100916	BRMS1L	0.949812	0.022362523	0.410967404
ENSG00000156983	BRPF1	0.889731	0.050741064	0.155759668
ENSG00000096070	BRPF3	0.868321	0.061319833	0.185953837
ENSG00000185658	BRWD1	0.945079	0.024531949	0.255344088
ENSG00000095564	BTAF1	0.981687	0.008026909	0.187872983
ENSG00000169679	BUB1	0.908692	0.041583425	0.402099964
ENSG00000158636	C11orf30	0.893262	0.049021365	0.211366737
ENSG00000170468	C14orf169	0.914416	0.038856104	0.173884964
ENSG00000258315	C17orf49	0.908051	0.041889771	0.037744055
ENSG00000099991	CABIN1	0.938558	0.027538956	0.167849882
ENSG00000142453	CARM1	0.942526	0.025706515	0.200099352
ENSG00000108468	CBX1	0.963965	0.015938624	0.231318155
ENSG00000173894	CBX2	0.967924	0.014158633	1.057958081

ENSG00000122565	CBX3	0.912348	0.039839245	0.268024869
ENSG00000141582	CBX4	0.995357	0.00202131	0.263415618
ENSG00000094916	CBX5	0.954527	0.020211867	0.493364157
ENSG00000183741	CBX6	0.994725	0.002297125	0.973117954
ENSG00000100307	CBX7	0.995391	0.002006158	0.588476653
ENSG00000141570	CBX8	0.974469	0.011231929	0.153556325
ENSG00000176476	CCDC101	0.932333	0.030428788	0.235741716
ENSG00000094804	CDC6	0.957613	0.018809834	0.404898577
ENSG00000134371	CDC73	0.896985	0.047214893	0.094258684
ENSG00000170312	CDK1	0.983696	0.007138954	0.342401017
ENSG00000059758	CDK17	0.951931	0.021394564	0.20452732
ENSG00000123374	CDK2	0.999387	0.00026652	0.187000335
ENSG00000250506	CDK3	0.998542	0.000633665	0.030683047
ENSG00000164885	CDK5	0.968997	0.013677585	0.232423485
ENSG00000134058	CDK7	0.89911	0.046187121	0.268092951
ENSG00000136807	CDK9	0.952662	0.021060957	0.176688666
ENSG00000153046	CDYL	0.949686	0.022419951	0.211500642
ENSG00000166446	CDYL2	0.995334	0.002031009	0.74480677
ENSG00000099954	CECR2	0.951573	0.021557719	1.572098966
ENSG00000145241	CENPC	0.979889	0.008823089	0.246328216
ENSG00000167670	CHAF1A	0.931624	0.030759304	0.214548416
ENSG00000159259	CHAF1B	0.969176	0.013597466	0.241410063
ENSG00000153922	CHD1	0.929663	0.031674651	0.260048516
ENSG00000131778	CHD1L	0.915562	0.038312094	0.142966105
ENSG00000173575	CHD2	0.882924	0.054076779	0.123364765
ENSG00000170004	CHD3	0.999271	0.000316717	0.30916383
ENSG00000111642	CHD4	0.86733	0.061815473	0.087319751
ENSG00000116254	CHD5	0.752097	0.123726415	0.57795284
ENSG00000124177	CHD6	0.979322	0.009074593	0.30850235
ENSG00000171316	CHD7	0.994301	0.002482162	0.434878941
ENSG00000100888	CHD8	0.880711	0.055166628	0.183651444
ENSG00000177200	CHD9	0.994779	0.002273313	0.241732482
ENSG00000149554	CHEK1	0.97588	0.01060378	0.307497165
ENSG00000104472	CHRAC1	0.964693	0.01561076	0.251451283
ENSG00000160679	CHTOP	0.902015	0.044786222	0.091421643
ENSG00000213341	CHUK	0.910855	0.040550719	0.115214649
ENSG00000138433	CIR1	0.846123	0.07256646	0.240084791
ENSG00000122966	CIT	0.969954	0.013248679	0.35475605
ENSG00000164442	CITED2	0.992682	0.003189933	0.803976226
ENSG00000179862	CITED4	0.996501	0.001522368	1.265059704
ENSG00000074201	CLNS1A	0.916542	0.037847669	0.402723254
ENSG00000134852	CLOCK	0.998927	0.000466055	0.344606445
ENSG00000148204	CRB2	0.144234	0.840931647	0.226218986
ENSG00000005339	CREBBP	0.930462	0.031301574	0.183128121

ENSG00000101266	CSNK2A1	0.88362	0.053734507	0.194601013
ENSG00000232838	CSRP2BP	0.986167	0.00604945	0.066345381
ENSG00000159692	CTBP1	0.945812	0.024195367	0.174885353
ENSG00000175029	CTBP2	0.932814	0.030204983	0.142774571
ENSG00000102974	CTCF	0.93813	0.027736774	0.073174019
ENSG00000124092	CTCFL	2.9E-05	4.537819095	0.920714244
ENSG00000198730	CTR9	0.865322	0.062822085	0.142262182
ENSG00000055130	CUL1	0.906138	0.042805586	0.173174595
ENSG00000108094	CUL2	0.881337	0.054857807	0.234414384
ENSG00000036257	CUL3	0.916471	0.037881468	0.211262104
ENSG00000139842	CUL4A	0.93158	0.030779958	0.400214702
ENSG00000166266	CUL5	0.985142	0.006501185	0.136914439
ENSG00000154832	CXXC1	0.937036	0.028243515	0.231344691
ENSG00000167657	DAPK3	0.942523	0.025708008	0.314456741
ENSG00000204209	DAXX	0.837469	0.077031091	0.096556487
ENSG00000167986	DDB1	0.855689	0.067684242	0.150276366
ENSG00000134574	DDB2	0.978742	0.009331628	0.206344086
ENSG00000165732	DDX21	0.985153	0.006496151	0.322487149
ENSG00000107625	DDX50	0.905656	0.043036919	0.104802381
ENSG00000124795	DEK	0.994232	0.002512314	0.257336557
ENSG00000101191	DIDO1	0.901365	0.045099295	0.183623308
ENSG00000178028	DMAP1	0.91809	0.037114636	0.175502694
ENSG00000136770	DNAJC1	0.979801	0.008862293	0.23742737
ENSG00000105821	DNAJC2	0.952965	0.020922913	0.315613943
ENSG00000130816	DNMT1	0.950887	0.021870871	0.239768869
ENSG00000119772	DNMT3A	0.951225	0.021716554	0.399215886
ENSG00000088305	DNMT3B	0.91003	0.040944255	0.530933716
ENSG00000142182	DNMT3L	0.002667	2.574031268	0.032739777
ENSG00000067334	DNTTIP2	0.898591	0.046437979	0.149753967
ENSG00000104885	DOT1L	0.861755	0.06461623	0.234084286
ENSG00000011332	DPF1	0.255378	0.592817125	0.667821713
ENSG00000133884	DPF2	0.91289	0.039581759	0.159673417
ENSG00000205683	DPF3	0.97542	0.010808157	0.113785407
ENSG00000187569	DPPA3	2.9E-05	4.537819095	0.029044448
ENSG00000162961	DPY30	0.958768	0.018286417	0.230576394
ENSG00000117505	DR1	0.900912	0.045317699	0.107256241
ENSG00000163840	DTX3L	0.992174	0.003412196	0.598622859
ENSG00000198919	DZIP3	0.989495	0.004586278	0.286371476
ENSG00000074266	EED	0.867876	0.061542128	0.167580537
ENSG00000181090	EHMT1	0.87184	0.059562965	0.157652324
ENSG00000204371	EHMT2	0.972805	0.011974174	0.185190348
ENSG00000255302	EID1	0.967565	0.014319752	0.24310809
ENSG00000176396	EID2	0.916937	0.037660532	0.124913597
ENSG00000176401	EID2B	0.991679	0.003628763	0.073266894

ENSG00000134759	ELP2	0.972382	0.012163222	0.311340653
ENSG00000134014	ELP3	0.817335	0.087599728	0.171278786
ENSG00000109911	ELP4	0.907029	0.042378991	0.185018043
ENSG00000170291	ELP5	0.940726	0.026536773	0.25199349
ENSG00000163832	ELP6	0.907882	0.041970596	0.086415305
ENSG00000120533	ENY2	0.876507	0.057244489	0.14986941
ENSG00000100393	EP300	0.868021	0.061469531	0.179616345
ENSG00000183495	EP400	0.938265	0.027674491	0.180343954
ENSG00000120616	EPC1	0.95042	0.022084301	0.142955552
ENSG00000135999	EPC2	0.910855	0.040550957	0.125841918
ENSG00000178568	ERBB4	0.651815	0.185875362	0.152161504
ENSG00000225830	ERCC6	0.896231	0.047579926	0.288132901
ENSG00000182150	ERCC6L2	0.934763	0.029298297	0.227691339
ENSG00000171311	EXOSC1	0.894507	0.048416137	0.16392744
ENSG00000130713	EXOSC2	0.971362	0.012618748	0.202163006
ENSG00000107371	EXOSC3	0.853582	0.068754947	0.251264347
ENSG00000178896	EXOSC4	0.947432	0.023452129	0.313977357
ENSG00000077348	EXOSC5	0.968308	0.013986308	0.295703188
ENSG00000223496	EXOSC6	0.953107	0.020858224	0.145587474
ENSG00000075914	EXOSC7	0.901379	0.045092415	0.164820777
ENSG00000120699	EXOSC8	0.882285	0.054390968	0.192937477
ENSG00000123737	EXOSC9	0.851444	0.06984411	0.148840282
ENSG00000104313	EYA1	0.66098	0.179811424	0.363435072
ENSG00000064655	EYA2	0.985365	0.006402982	2.161665549
ENSG00000158161	EYA3	0.912117	0.039949394	0.208946587
ENSG00000112319	EYA4	0.840365	0.075532177	0.979743423
ENSG00000108799	EZH1	0.980246	0.008664754	0.199792801
ENSG00000106462	EZH2	0.989136	0.004743832	0.248729592
ENSG00000163322	FAM175A	0.983002	0.007445784	0.111354073
ENSG00000165660	FAM175B	0.945061	0.02454034	0.10889553
ENSG00000115392	FANCL	0.948051	0.023168431	0.15414585
ENSG00000105202	FBL	0.957362	0.018923831	0.312371098
ENSG00000156860	FBRS	0.894902	0.048224397	0.219208359
ENSG00000112787	FBRSL1	0.94003	0.026858167	0.283047064
ENSG00000147912	FBXO10	0.964644	0.015632717	0.137275689
ENSG00000138081	FBXO11	0.924977	0.03386889	0.14123107
ENSG00000092140	G2E3	0.882622	0.054225039	0.289354317
ENSG00000116717	GADD45A	0.984551	0.006761904	0.504130261
ENSG00000099860	GADD45B	0.999884	5.03559E-05	0.79744246
ENSG00000130222	GADD45G	0.971297	0.012647893	0.465391484
ENSG00000157259	GATAD1	0.955348	0.01983848	0.461517807
ENSG00000167491	GATAD2A	0.91769	0.037304015	0.167660027
ENSG00000143614	GATAD2B	0.870261	0.060350544	0.119562571
ENSG00000162676	GFI1	0.942082	0.025911263	0.327568565

ENSG00000165702	GFI1B	0.005689	2.244992866	0.021832998
ENSG00000140632	GLYR1	0.892903	0.049195846	0.122557717
ENSG00000131149	GSE1	0.994338	0.002466164	0.324779487
ENSG00000177602	GSG2	0.707068	0.150539021	0.25040269
ENSG00000263001	GTF2I	0.981594	0.008068015	0.269536847
ENSG00000125484	GTF3C4	0.99358	0.002796966	0.248792429
ENSG00000128708	HAT1	0.925414	0.033663883	0.231486281
ENSG00000111727	HCFC2	0.991088	0.003887638	0.205358702
ENSG00000116478	HDAC1	0.987987	0.005248628	0.260595013
ENSG00000100429	HDAC10	0.976029	0.010537285	0.225262353
ENSG00000163517	HDAC11	0.998107	0.000822787	0.274221045
ENSG00000196591	HDAC2	0.93376	0.029764793	0.1844794
ENSG00000171720	HDAC3	0.901638	0.044967947	0.149323859
ENSG00000068024	HDAC4	0.964439	0.015725156	0.432205859
ENSG00000108840	HDAC5	0.948894	0.022782229	0.269885493
ENSG00000061273	HDAC7	0.995956	0.00175995	0.192126761
ENSG00000048052	HDAC9	0.955198	0.019906792	1.144368808
ENSG00000143321	HDGF	0.976913	0.010144092	0.214101228
ENSG00000112273	HDGFL1	6.06E-05	4.217483944	0.093628577
ENSG00000167674	HDGFRP2	0.874491	0.058244647	0.134010011
ENSG00000166503	HDGFRP3	0.955918	0.019579194	0.410735768
ENSG00000119969	HELLS	0.899244	0.046122659	0.36529323
ENSG00000166135	HIF1AN	0.893605	0.048854494	0.131688055
ENSG00000172273	HINFP	0.883691	0.053699383	0.127335286
ENSG00000100084	HIRA	0.9347	0.029327897	0.128968591
ENSG00000149929	HIRIP3	0.862965	0.064006715	0.15765158
ENSG00000123485	HJURP	0.675398	0.170439911	0.434973563
ENSG00000159267	HLCS	0.969795	0.013320081	0.209423473
ENSG00000071794	HLTF	0.988202	0.005154319	0.612955097
ENSG00000140382	HMG20A	0.892413	0.049433991	0.083067877
ENSG00000064961	HMG20B	0.982393	0.007714901	0.295579231
ENSG00000189403	HMGB1	0.955043	0.019976857	0.233365781
ENSG00000205581	HMGN1	0.994675	0.002318746	0.235246167
ENSG00000198830	HMGN2	0.901555	0.045007673	0.307828863
ENSG00000118418	HMGN3	0.998738	0.000548352	0.390623007
ENSG00000182952	HMGN4	0.982607	0.007620308	0.114065661
ENSG00000127483	HP1BP3	0.912754	0.039646434	0.138584725
ENSG00000168453	HR	0.959757	0.017838785	1.567875799
ENSG00000169087	HSPBAP1	0.916196	0.038011457	0.208870807
ENSG00000070061	IKBKAP	0.951136	0.021757542	0.188911119
ENSG00000185811	IKZF1	0.973435	0.011693199	0.570784006
ENSG00000161405	IKZF3	0.914045	0.039032207	1.049831636
ENSG00000153487	ING1	0.949415	0.022543735	0.140110214
ENSG00000168556	ING2	0.965785	0.01511932	0.151304752

ENSG00000071243	ING3	0.93242	0.030388285	0.115143337
ENSG00000111653	ING4	0.923962	0.034345906	0.202254998
ENSG00000168395	ING5	0.92694	0.032948347	0.161848385
ENSG00000128908	INO80	0.893848	0.048736092	0.105839644
ENSG00000115274	INO80B	0.916192	0.03801355	0.15878986
ENSG00000153391	INO80C	0.96041	0.017543175	0.373467896
ENSG00000114933	INO80D	0.974275	0.01131828	0.250287255
ENSG00000169592	INO80E	0.944596	0.024753953	0.166011904
ENSG00000138785	INTS12	0.913267	0.039402008	0.114637884
ENSG00000077684	JADE1	0.96013	0.017669764	0.323660386
ENSG00000043143	JADE2	0.980284	0.008647926	1.11642394
ENSG00000096968	JAK2	0.963258	0.016257567	0.521166433
ENSG00000008083	JARID2	0.938697	0.027474562	0.333307361
ENSG00000140044	JDP2	0.999333	0.000289626	0.363768493
ENSG00000171988	JMJD1C	0.88142	0.054816956	0.342742286
ENSG00000081692	JMJD4	0.967117	0.01452093	0.176694654
ENSG00000070495	JMJD6	0.928003	0.032450608	0.144471672
ENSG00000243789	JMJD7	0.940238	0.026762331	0.070076496
ENSG00000161999	JMJD8	0.940967	0.026425737	0.221532548
ENSG00000120071	KANSL1	0.901617	0.044977707	0.10363127
ENSG00000139620	KANSL2	0.788276	0.103321772	0.132316364
ENSG00000114982	KANSL3	0.855742	0.067657087	0.129993675
ENSG00000108773	KAT2A	0.979322	0.009074593	0.190854345
ENSG00000114166	KAT2B	0.99987	5.66508E-05	0.823028909
ENSG00000172977	KAT5	0.927188	0.032832201	0.127847595
ENSG00000083168	KAT6A	0.930215	0.031416482	0.531084699
ENSG00000156650	KAT6B	0.993091	0.003010743	0.155464667
ENSG00000136504	KAT7	0.915071	0.038545165	0.112724765
ENSG00000103510	KAT8	0.861398	0.064795891	0.121097688
ENSG00000004487	KDM1A	0.907397	0.042202433	0.234503199
ENSG00000165097	KDM1B	0.924393	0.034143444	0.323021577
ENSG00000173120	KDM2A	0.953626	0.020621747	0.226171818
ENSG00000089094	KDM2B	0.901788	0.044895311	0.140674467
ENSG00000115548	KDM3A	0.932496	0.030352999	0.272751641
ENSG00000120733	KDM3B	0.94812	0.023136663	0.130864899
ENSG00000066135	KDM4A	0.973841	0.011512132	0.192091503
ENSG00000127663	KDM4B	0.913238	0.039416255	0.223405303
ENSG00000107077	KDM4C	0.915029	0.038565149	0.214085413
ENSG00000186280	KDM4D	0.940165	0.026795959	0.064435751
ENSG00000235268	KDM4E	0.039819	1.399909602	0.015681364
ENSG00000073614	KDM5A	0.980721	0.008454588	0.246173139
ENSG00000117139	KDM5B	0.974675	0.01114012	0.35692669
ENSG00000132510	KDM6B	0.956471	0.01932838	0.281677094
ENSG00000006459	KDM7A	0.990385	0.004196115	0.61222643

ENSG00000155666	KDM8	0.947413	0.023460656	0.065658003
ENSG00000079999	KEAP1	0.927942	0.032479154	0.285967235
ENSG00000118058	KMT2A	0.935971	0.0287376	0.198421341
ENSG00000272333	KMT2B	0.929601	0.031703312	0.245355279
ENSG00000055609	KMT2C	0.906275	0.042740235	0.329944147
ENSG00000167548	KMT2D	0.879877	0.055577886	0.260766417
ENSG00000005483	KMT2E	0.950072	0.022243269	0.321897773
ENSG00000185513	L3MBTL1	0.959842	0.017800128	0.446632928
ENSG00000100395	L3MBTL2	0.887005	0.052074158	0.067690212
ENSG00000198945	L3MBTL3	0.961933	0.016854978	0.164706737
ENSG00000154655	L3MBTL4	0.955052	0.019972766	0.805128074
ENSG00000143815	LBR	0.974446	0.011242154	0.364829746
ENSG00000166477	LEO1	0.887188	0.051984121	0.209673607
ENSG00000161036	LRWD1	0.935461	0.028974118	0.244922293
ENSG00000135341	MAP3K7	0.881522	0.054766973	0.150206179
ENSG00000114738	MAPKAPK3	0.967074	0.014540335	0.398557706
ENSG00000120539	MASTL	0.936545	0.028471273	0.258117754
ENSG00000141644	MBD1	0.826581	0.082714614	0.300487226
ENSG00000134046	MBD2	0.934847	0.029259635	0.328089953
ENSG00000071655	MBD3	0.899279	0.046105413	0.254115839
ENSG00000129071	MBD4	0.914406	0.038861029	0.197409402
ENSG00000204406	MBD5	0.947204	0.023556572	0.232327826
ENSG00000166987	MBD6	0.982009	0.007884442	0.11569223
ENSG00000151332	MBIP	0.997886	0.000918881	0.306511232
ENSG00000011258	MBTD1	0.933033	0.030103154	0.217953673
ENSG00000187778	MCRS1	0.890851	0.050194897	0.148282798
ENSG00000137337	MDC1	0.952744	0.021023559	0.212890727
ENSG00000163875	MEAF6	0.806782	0.093243824	0.154912841
ENSG00000133895	MEN1	0.957718	0.018762392	0.188069615
ENSG00000174197	MGA	0.939353	0.027171029	0.136616478
ENSG00000198408	MGEA5	0.938308	0.027654723	0.157246681
ENSG00000170430	MGMT	0.923939	0.034356516	0.623104449
ENSG00000170854	MINA	0.975205	0.01090406	0.227430856
ENSG00000130382	MLLT1	0.950435	0.022077678	0.189632548
ENSG00000078403	MLLT10	0.981167	0.008256982	0.155377726
ENSG00000275023	MLLT6	0.973586	0.011625636	0.258626122
ENSG00000159256	MORC3	0.904508	0.043587735	0.253455739
ENSG00000185787	MORF4L1	0.95752	0.018852317	0.097433354
ENSG00000155363	MOV10	0.99683	0.001378714	0.354451013
ENSG00000196199	MPHOSPH8	0.936232	0.028616573	0.208927355
ENSG00000101189	MRGBP	0.812236	0.090317953	0.237812703
ENSG00000116062	MSH6	0.907605	0.042103131	0.254106981
ENSG00000188895	MSL1	0.866862	0.062050266	0.087082146
ENSG00000174579	MSL2	0.878195	0.056408798	0.303734181

ENSG00000173531	MST1	0.983788	0.007098639	0.136654148
ENSG00000182979	MTA1	0.923044	0.034777519	0.23861737
ENSG00000149480	MTA2	0.944184	0.024943439	0.128335913
ENSG00000057935	MTA3	0.999338	0.000287798	0.177484734
ENSG00000137265	MUM1	0.902172	0.044710682	0.442360597
ENSG00000132382	MYBBP1A	0.924416	0.034132357	0.292546256
ENSG00000197879	MYO1C	0.999653	0.000150728	0.330068973
ENSG00000162601	MYSM1	0.972406	0.012152461	0.34292449
ENSG00000122390	NAA60	0.913649	0.039220784	0.115155279
ENSG00000187109	NAP1L1	0.978878	0.009271274	0.205569547
ENSG00000205531	NAP1L4	0.880393	0.05532325	0.185211488
ENSG00000177432	NAP1L5	0.994511	0.002390391	0.283462369
ENSG00000132780	NASP	0.929529	0.031737036	0.280428967
ENSG00000135372	NAT10	0.868249	0.061355957	0.252771394
ENSG00000104320	NBN	0.923754	0.034443845	0.21509323
ENSG00000115053	NCL	0.893183	0.049059793	0.232281202
ENSG00000084676	NCOA1	0.961714	0.016953933	0.291434478
ENSG00000140396	NCOA2	0.906028	0.042858257	0.342475687
ENSG00000124151	NCOA3	0.983436	0.007254082	0.467818406
ENSG00000198646	NCOA6	0.818055	0.08721765	0.140309811
ENSG00000141027	NCOR1	0.826244	0.0828915	0.247398306
ENSG00000196498	NCOR2	0.95858	0.018371768	0.268004693
ENSG00000119408	NEK6	0.964909	0.015513602	0.570637374
ENSG00000119638	NEK9	0.917171	0.037549708	0.205845771
ENSG00000170322	NFRKB	0.965194	0.015385206	0.263346058
ENSG00000120837	NFYB	0.899501	0.045998467	0.133562227
ENSG00000066136	NFYC	0.899742	0.045881801	0.309698266
ENSG00000164190	NIPBL	0.907653	0.042079974	0.306936002
ENSG00000188976	NOC2L	0.853055	0.069023114	0.276883381
ENSG00000170485	NPAS2	0.966869	0.014632229	0.900640074
ENSG00000181163	NPM1	0.93592	0.028761158	0.317917417
ENSG00000158806	NPM2	0.952338	0.021208951	0.304263843
ENSG00000165671	NSD1	0.84803	0.071588745	0.25545226
ENSG00000117697	NSL1	0.935885	0.028777503	0.130506273
ENSG00000142623	PADI1	0.043174	1.364778588	2.923343179
ENSG00000117115	PADI2	0.928962	0.032001861	1.724201252
ENSG00000142619	PADI3	0.024103	1.617936753	2.947543151
ENSG00000159339	PADI4	0.733116	0.134827336	0.05279436
ENSG00000006712	PAF1	0.886358	0.052390867	0.175935408
ENSG00000280789	PAGR1	0.953116	0.020854017	0.111751308
ENSG00000180370	PAK2	0.959076	0.018147086	0.260173229
ENSG00000083093	PALB2	0.929826	0.031598081	0.128821865
ENSG00000227345	PARG	0.871639	0.059663298	0.135205068
ENSG00000143799	PARP1	0.909213	0.041334214	0.250210995

ENSG00000129484	PARP2	0.999653	0.000150728	0.179973262
ENSG00000041880	PARP3	0.984553	0.006761081	0.452588319
ENSG00000157212	PAXIP1	0.956909	0.01912958	0.209901389
ENSG00000168078	PBK	0.542821	0.265343749	0.466399449
ENSG00000163939	PBRM1	0.94204	0.025930713	0.202339566
ENSG00000115289	PCGF1	0.853055	0.069023114	0.192733052
ENSG00000277258	PCGF2	0.972044	0.012313909	0.215151075
ENSG00000185619	PCGF3	0.964517	0.015690275	0.241933248
ENSG00000180628	PCGF5	0.899486	0.046005396	0.244951382
ENSG00000156374	PCGF6	0.995442	0.001984196	0.087436821
ENSG00000132646	PCNA	0.892142	0.049566122	0.4361057
ENSG00000164951	PDP1	0.986919	0.0057183	0.59487692
ENSG00000141456	PELP1	0.875174	0.057905604	0.214412834
ENSG00000111752	PHC1	0.990932	0.003956116	0.316953679
ENSG00000134686	PHC2	0.941634	0.02611792	0.274144266
ENSG00000173889	PHC3	0.961365	0.017111679	0.407493574
ENSG00000112511	PHF1	0.955613	0.019718084	0.155538611
ENSG00000130024	PHF10	0.991278	0.003804706	0.195323315
ENSG00000136147	PHF11	0.979522	0.008985921	0.322707536
ENSG00000109118	PHF12	0.899222	0.046132886	0.132020709
ENSG00000116273	PHF13	0.925966	0.033404839	0.189227988
ENSG00000106443	PHF14	0.950915	0.021858381	0.28330921
ENSG00000119403	PHF19	0.993485	0.002838648	0.349128432
ENSG00000197724	PHF2	0.949348	0.02257464	0.186659705
ENSG00000025293	PHF20	0.976782	0.010202446	0.180757662
ENSG00000129292	PHF20L1	0.872118	0.059424748	0.17306851
ENSG00000135365	PHF21A	0.943422	0.025293866	0.188557763
ENSG00000056487	PHF21B	0.76418	0.116804076	0.140908156
ENSG00000040633	PHF23	0.927345	0.032758478	0.18378419
ENSG00000118482	PHF3	0.878421	0.056297264	0.188891215
ENSG00000100410	PHF5A	0.859468	0.065770245	0.12196699
ENSG00000010318	PHF7	0.929301	0.031843637	0.100949249
ENSG00000146247	PHIP	0.942686	0.025633116	0.198806001
ENSG00000070047	PHRF1	0.821748	0.085261492	0.194658076
ENSG00000134627	PIWIL4	0.977323	0.009961846	0.127185527
ENSG00000067225	PKM	0.966546	0.014777332	0.453582255
ENSG00000123143	PKN1	0.997625	0.001032759	0.866612584
ENSG00000143442	POGZ	0.921125	0.035681337	0.175517148
ENSG00000148229	POLE3	0.975758	0.010658068	0.272247162
ENSG00000109819	PPARGC1A	0.969878	0.013282704	1.440828586
ENSG00000115241	PPM1G	0.895745	0.047815762	0.205795942
ENSG00000113575	PPP2CA	0.908936	0.041466614	0.253834643
ENSG00000149923	PPP4C	0.924742	0.033979586	0.278273836
ENSG00000163605	PPP4R2	0.875749	0.057620417	0.167443239

ENSG00000100796	PPP4R3A	0.916831	0.03771082	0.182556042
ENSG00000275052	PPP4R3B	0.916905	0.037675596	0.087073217
ENSG00000057657	PRDM1	0.987987	0.005248628	1.000890154
ENSG00000170325	PRDM10	0.927418	0.032724315	0.077628597
ENSG00000019485	PRDM11	0.977072	0.010073226	0.23715169
ENSG00000130711	PRDM12	0.007275	2.138145374	0.039743604
ENSG00000112238	PRDM13	2.9E-05	4.537819095	0.17317427
ENSG00000147596	PRDM14	2.9E-05	4.537819095	0.043707827
ENSG00000141956	PRDM15	0.878037	0.056487277	0.065388735
ENSG00000142611	PRDM16	0.961909	0.016865971	0.447648225
ENSG00000116731	PRDM2	0.953302	0.020769615	0.200227791
ENSG00000110851	PRDM4	0.925908	0.033431989	0.150222202
ENSG00000138738	PRDM5	0.957892	0.018683347	0.304829523
ENSG00000061455	PRDM6	0.909288	0.041298598	0.213223988
ENSG00000126856	PRDM7	2.9E-05	4.537819095	0.020305176
ENSG00000152784	PRDM8	0.976938	0.010132792	0.317708251
ENSG00000164256	PRDM9	2.9E-05	4.537819095	0.079954816
ENSG00000132356	PRKAA1	0.956727	0.019211846	0.38497567
ENSG00000162409	PRKAA2	0.97292	0.01192295	1.284864947
ENSG00000111725	PRKAB1	0.927061	0.032891851	0.213170316
ENSG00000131791	PRKAB2	0.993722	0.002734922	0.271318198
ENSG00000181929	PRKAG1	0.913404	0.039336969	0.197431833
ENSG00000106617	PRKAG2	0.956415	0.019353447	0.266339103
ENSG00000115592	PRKAG3	3.17E-05	4.498999364	0.038038798
ENSG00000154229	PRKCA	0.988406	0.005064716	0.744887578
ENSG00000166501	PRKCB	0.978556	0.009414213	0.61517762
ENSG00000163932	PRKCD	0.985769	0.00622501	0.292460743
ENSG00000253729	PRKDC	0.902322	0.044638321	0.39373434
ENSG00000126457	PRMT1	0.84928	0.070948919	0.241027417
ENSG00000160310	PRMT2	0.976101	0.010505053	0.250895295
ENSG00000185238	PRMT3	0.966735	0.014692551	0.223306015
ENSG00000100462	PRMT5	0.903549	0.044048352	0.243978115
ENSG00000198890	PRMT6	0.996228	0.001641165	0.248504686
ENSG00000132600	PRMT7	0.932769	0.030225681	0.280248689
ENSG00000111218	PRMT8	0.043609	1.360423647	0.182774382
ENSG00000164169	PRMT9	0.895113	0.048122241	0.127489154
ENSG00000105618	PRPF31	0.796183	0.098987299	0.14932102
ENSG00000156858	PRR14	0.954501	0.020223707	0.155405662
ENSG00000164985	PSIP1	0.948531	0.02294856	0.437261518
ENSG00000171813	PWWP2B	0.963823	0.016002685	0.235716927
ENSG00000171016	PYGO1	0.955204	0.01990376	0.944486915
ENSG00000163348	PYGO2	0.895038	0.048158612	0.116944216
ENSG00000051180	RAD51	0.945495	0.024340536	0.280872264
ENSG00000197275	RAD54B	0.932844	0.030190896	0.113037863

ENSG00000085999	RAD54L	0.942868	0.025549164	0.261058668
ENSG00000164080	RAD54L2	0.870252	0.060354787	0.191906888
ENSG00000166349	RAG1	0.750106	0.124877139	0.656617511
ENSG00000175097	RAG2	0.00229	2.640192004	0.020484916
ENSG00000108557	RAI1	0.988249	0.005133524	0.278529582
ENSG00000139687	RB1	0.934159	0.029579002	0.475854318
ENSG00000162521	RBBP4	0.805779	0.093783989	0.225550365
ENSG00000117222	RBBP5	0.87218	0.059393652	0.106589833
ENSG00000100387	RBX1	0.943108	0.025438424	0.20583828
ENSG00000180198	RCC1	0.978221	0.009563081	0.328301531
ENSG00000089902	RCOR1	0.955767	0.019648027	0.487411287
ENSG00000117625	RCOR3	0.877474	0.056765899	0.176571327
ENSG00000084093	REST	0.995712	0.001866206	0.135435323
ENSG00000204227	RING1	0.867813	0.061573851	0.155572682
ENSG00000178966	RMI1	0.946647	0.023812155	0.257067248
ENSG00000163961	RNF168	0.959636	0.017893304	0.470413727
ENSG00000121481	RNF2	0.891098	0.050074656	0.123627193
ENSG00000155827	RNF20	0.901343	0.04511	0.138888533
ENSG00000103549	RNF40	0.886973	0.052089571	0.161282517
ENSG00000112130	RNF8	0.896406	0.047495238	0.110245165
ENSG00000162302	RPS6KA4	0.996261	0.001626927	0.446114833
ENSG00000100784	RPS6KA5	0.917348	0.037465964	0.41424836
ENSG00000132275	RRP8	0.880106	0.055464988	0.089560607
ENSG00000048649	RSF1	0.897962	0.046742	0.19565862
ENSG00000175792	RUVBL1	0.854148	0.068466967	0.330337019
ENSG00000183207	RUVBL2	0.866727	0.062117675	0.18707928
ENSG00000163602	RYBP	0.962631	0.016540272	0.205643011
ENSG00000160633	SAFB	0.818369	0.087050708	0.058102016
ENSG00000136715	SAP130	0.803228	0.095161294	0.127836861
ENSG00000150459	SAP18	0.839605	0.075925055	0.255306194
ENSG00000205307	SAP25	0.985055	0.006539314	0.02738678
ENSG00000164105	SAP30	0.948807	0.022822162	0.199469808
ENSG00000164576	SAP30L	0.945061	0.02454034	0.176845532
ENSG00000182568	SATB1	0.998	0.000869459	0.413680075
ENSG00000119042	SATB2	0.976152	0.010482767	0.35911944
ENSG00000010803	SCMH1	0.997681	0.00100813	0.404258582
ENSG00000146285	SCML4	0.854955	0.068056905	0.116816539
ENSG00000079387	SENP1	0.923712	0.034463576	0.131543084
ENSG00000161956	SENP3	0.863964	0.063504372	0.154139329
ENSG00000119335	SET	0.961725	0.016949258	0.243500099
ENSG00000099381	SETD1A	0.894984	0.048184618	0.086848509
ENSG00000139718	SETD1B	0.943236	0.025379542	0.161523211
ENSG00000181555	SETD2	0.836423	0.077574025	0.170950993
ENSG00000183576	SETD3	0.941094	0.026366892	0.210605281

ENSG00000185917	SETD4	0.917353	0.037463322	0.169858771
ENSG00000168137	SETD5	0.919087	0.036643397	0.216948622
ENSG00000103037	SETD6	0.995426	0.001991078	0.208983061
ENSG00000145391	SETD7	0.999653	0.000150728	0.223798221
ENSG00000183955	SETD8	0.954928	0.020029583	0.185194168
ENSG00000155542	SETD9	0.938318	0.027649868	0.215670632
ENSG00000143379	SETDB1	0.922084	0.035229523	0.148350183
ENSG00000136169	SETDB2	0.978922	0.009251758	0.109089498
ENSG00000170364	SETMAR	0.999637	0.00015758	0.241785595
ENSG00000115524	SF3B1	0.955232	0.01989119	0.133746397
ENSG00000189091	SF3B3	0.885435	0.052843422	0.188533079
ENSG00000163935	SFMBT1	0.986869	0.005740361	0.185611828
ENSG00000198879	SFMBT2	0.974834	0.011069277	0.531919708
ENSG00000116560	SFPQ	0.843218	0.074060108	0.072273906
ENSG00000146414	SHPRH	0.919542	0.036428494	0.156371039
ENSG00000169375	SIN3A	0.910429	0.040753703	0.094315673
ENSG00000127511	SIN3B	0.938399	0.027612294	0.135421005
ENSG00000096717	SIRT1	0.889242	0.050979826	0.159170479
ENSG00000068903	SIRT2	0.879819	0.055606661	0.276398422
ENSG00000142082	SIRT3	0.924872	0.033918284	0.117107846
ENSG00000089163	SIRT4	0.979397	0.009041372	0.11407281
ENSG00000124523	SIRT5	0.915801	0.038199074	0.150593592
ENSG00000077463	SIRT6	0.941449	0.026203075	0.196186977
ENSG00000187531	SIRT7	0.958771	0.018284937	0.342473552
ENSG00000113558	SKP1	0.945243	0.024456379	0.200475927
ENSG00000133302	SLF1	0.929173	0.03190345	0.130828408
ENSG00000080503	SMARCA2	0.928081	0.032414137	0.567940511
ENSG00000127616	SMARCA4	0.892385	0.049447512	0.229322393
ENSG00000153147	SMARCA5	0.915234	0.038467621	0.163366616
ENSG00000163104	SMARCAD1	0.997918	0.000905152	0.177794974
ENSG00000138375	SMARCAL1	0.866722	0.062120278	0.119802763
ENSG00000099956	SMARCB1	0.850823	0.070160598	0.198616371
ENSG00000173473	SMARCC1	0.933262	0.029996632	0.148954713
ENSG00000139613	SMARCC2	0.935371	0.029015984	0.11140078
ENSG00000066117	SMARCD1	0.925721	0.033519848	0.163924606
ENSG00000108604	SMARCD2	0.963962	0.015940102	0.206535504
ENSG00000082014	SMARCD3	0.964599	0.015653151	0.683600861
ENSG00000073584	SMARCE1	0.910348	0.040792326	0.176538132
ENSG00000115593	SMYD1	0.166893	0.77756211	0.095259635
ENSG00000143499	SMYD2	0.970618	0.012951479	0.164209154
ENSG00000185420	SMYD3	0.926772	0.033027203	0.265503925
ENSG00000186532	SMYD4	0.872003	0.059481944	0.133018736
ENSG00000135632	SMYD5	0.922981	0.034807205	0.162222373
ENSG00000067066	SP100	0.998174	0.000793784	0.423358723

ENSG00000135899	SP110	0.997449	0.001109181	0.430432345
ENSG00000079263	SP140	0.936632	0.028431204	0.413353859
ENSG00000185404	SP140L	0.998865	0.000493191	0.462681509
ENSG00000065526	SPEN	0.919508	0.036444633	0.163483668
ENSG00000121067	SPOP	0.977217	0.010008813	0.113713111
ENSG00000080603	SRCAP	0.855279	0.067892174	0.119025765
ENSG00000136450	SRSF1	0.946174	0.02402903	0.081568496
ENSG00000112081	SRSF3	0.925174	0.033776621	0.087277734
ENSG00000184402	SS18L1	0.972713	0.012015309	0.166648979
ENSG00000008324	SS18L2	0.946319	0.023962513	0.130796204
ENSG00000149136	SSRP1	0.887621	0.051772662	0.187206093
ENSG00000101109	STK4	0.969762	0.013334711	0.168338756
ENSG00000111707	SUDS3	0.885975	0.052578707	0.154006064
ENSG00000092201	SUPT16H	0.886856	0.052146774	0.229601953
ENSG00000196284	SUPT3H	0.948938	0.022762073	0.188843335
ENSG00000109111	SUPT6H	0.874841	0.05807108	0.116681291
ENSG00000119760	SUPT7L	0.925809	0.033478424	0.075011988
ENSG00000152455	SUV39H2	0.96071	0.017407789	0.145100692
ENSG00000110066	SUV420H1	0.910763	0.040594395	0.2834373
ENSG00000133247	SUV420H2	0.968241	0.014016582	0.208239202
ENSG00000178691	SUZ12	0.853803	0.068642308	0.173951884
ENSG00000135316	SYNCRIP	0.934864	0.029251733	0.141961242
ENSG00000152382	TADA1	0.979905	0.008815866	0.084326295
ENSG00000276234	TADA2A	0.884938	0.053086929	0.126444263
ENSG00000173011	TADA2B	0.939608	0.027053367	0.188469434
ENSG00000171148	TADA3	0.927912	0.03249309	0.248168311
ENSG00000166337	TAF10	0.940137	0.026808957	0.376416501
ENSG00000120656	TAF12	0.88721	0.051973742	0.26324257
ENSG00000122728	TAF1L	2.9E-05	4.537819095	0.037541646
ENSG00000064313	TAF2	0.859414	0.065797763	0.160498606
ENSG00000165632	TAF3	0.870212	0.060374872	0.188373044
ENSG00000130699	TAF4	0.933312	0.029973009	0.123863272
ENSG00000148835	TAF5	0.932569	0.030318918	0.102308163
ENSG00000135801	TAF5L	0.934732	0.029312954	0.093960065
ENSG00000106290	TAF6	0.931943	0.03061059	0.267665563
ENSG00000162227	TAF6L	0.919186	0.036596826	0.132132779
ENSG00000178913	TAF7	0.883003	0.054037819	0.208941728
ENSG00000137413	TAF8	0.935414	0.028996083	0.128169578
ENSG00000273841	TAF9	0.935234	0.029079812	0.252432891
ENSG00000177565	TBL1XR1	0.96542	0.015283578	0.350456878
ENSG00000139372	TDG	0.972522	0.012100682	0.173453454
ENSG00000083544	TDRD3	0.958107	0.018585871	0.120958686
ENSG00000196116	TDRD7	0.932964	0.030135323	0.393961252
ENSG00000182134	TDRKH	0.985365	0.006402982	0.448856833

ENSG00000138336	TET1	0.933855	0.029720518	0.493405074
ENSG00000168769	TET2	0.997899	0.000913608	0.397908238
ENSG00000187605	TET3	0.969191	0.013590497	0.450995304
ENSG00000136891	TEX10	0.884085	0.053505893	0.174904865
ENSG00000198176	TFDP1	0.93124	0.03093829	0.443826479
ENSG00000105619	TFPT	0.917033	0.037615051	0.148107309
ENSG00000196781	TLE1	0.972413	0.012149132	0.525746344
ENSG00000065717	TLE2	0.941043	0.026390691	0.879426052
ENSG00000106829	TLE4	0.994897	0.002221741	0.647016832
ENSG00000198586	TLK1	0.908954	0.041458075	0.251462423
ENSG00000146872	TLK2	0.843501	0.073914509	0.074928405
ENSG00000118245	TNP1	0.556752	0.254338308	0.002961072
ENSG00000178279	TNP2	2.9E-05	4.537819095	0.014324435
ENSG00000160949	TONSL	0.998843	0.000502723	0.313179946
ENSG00000131747	TOP2A	0.926216	0.033287812	0.609530209
ENSG00000077097	TOP2B	0.950435	0.022077678	0.34914505
ENSG00000067369	TP53BP1	0.973533	0.011649268	0.177699681
ENSG00000221926	TRIM16	0.963155	0.016304009	0.796032768
ENSG00000122779	TRIM24	0.939833	0.026949156	0.378508252
ENSG00000204713	TRIM27	0.944768	0.024674772	0.193827096
ENSG00000130726	TRIM28	0.897408	0.047010075	0.414717351
ENSG00000197323	TRIM33	0.916501	0.037867162	0.227890096
ENSG00000166436	TRIM66	0.978103	0.009615567	0.28135805
ENSG00000196367	TRRAP	0.848692	0.07125003	0.378324538
ENSG00000178093	TSSK6	0.975674	0.010695475	0.074784271
ENSG00000112742	TTK	0.590767	0.228583833	0.333311978
ENSG00000162971	TYW5	0.923582	0.03452472	0.105626328
ENSG00000119048	UBE2B	0.886562	0.052291102	0.256285841
ENSG00000072401	UBE2D1	0.980536	0.008536354	0.213779562
ENSG00000109332	UBE2D3	0.949841	0.02234928	0.196226309
ENSG00000170142	UBE2E1	0.912803	0.039622927	0.196590187
ENSG00000186591	UBE2H	0.905	0.043351421	0.286892757
ENSG00000177889	UBE2N	0.89997	0.045772047	0.125791613
ENSG00000077152	UBE2T	0.995793	0.001831027	0.324178444
ENSG00000118900	UBN1	0.915767	0.038215072	0.162625931
ENSG00000024048	UBR2	0.963348	0.016216878	0.240409409
ENSG00000104517	UBR5	0.931264	0.030927268	0.241920118
ENSG00000012963	UBR7	0.873258	0.058857638	0.167412017
ENSG00000116750	UCHL5	0.940217	0.02677172	0.127775453
ENSG00000276043	UHRF1	0.876306	0.057344063	0.37278028
ENSG00000147854	UHRF2	0.911073	0.040446778	0.284099137
ENSG00000087206	UIMC1	0.94592	0.024145479	0.133596631
ENSG00000152484	USP12	0.934058	0.029626169	0.275692479
ENSG00000135655	USP15	0.957899	0.018680383	0.231157292

ENSG00000156256	USP16	0.93224	0.030472384	0.152507107
ENSG00000223443	USP17L2	1	0	0.013673239
ENSG00000143258	USP21	0.882617	0.054227591	0.204012
ENSG00000124422	USP22	0.946478	0.023889357	0.304939687
ENSG00000140455	USP3	0.954435	0.020253742	0.133224172
ENSG00000055483	USP36	0.915638	0.038276343	0.150126236
ENSG00000136014	USP44	0.945401	0.024383985	0.136463766
ENSG00000109189	USP46	0.916496	0.037869312	0.338157186
ENSG00000164663	USP49	0.905714	0.043008782	0.220008781
ENSG00000187555	USP7	0.86209	0.064447279	0.122187155
ENSG00000163159	VPS72	0.843128	0.074106581	0.165295966
ENSG00000100749	VRK1	0.928436	0.032248019	0.251548745
ENSG00000095787	WAC	0.832	0.079876674	0.129985999
ENSG00000196363	WDR5	0.883859	0.053617081	0.278605967
ENSG00000116455	WDR77	0.907705	0.042055192	0.210495621
ENSG00000164091	WDR82	0.915699	0.038247456	0.118328411
ENSG00000109685	WHSC1	0.927964	0.032469094	0.369098534
ENSG00000147548	WHSC1L1	0.986435	0.005931623	0.454849641
ENSG00000176871	WSB2	0.967449	0.014371796	0.260109175
ENSG00000015153	YAF2	0.912451	0.039790528	0.11846489
ENSG00000163872	YEATS2	0.949984	0.02228364	0.415095631
ENSG00000127337	YEATS4	0.874309	0.058334897	0.411556712
ENSG00000166913	YWHAB	0.978493	0.009442386	0.157961563
ENSG00000108953	YWHAE	0.895787	0.047795193	0.199563121
ENSG00000164924	YWHAZ	0.965214	0.015376412	0.492392851
ENSG00000078487	ZCWPW1	0.903138	0.044245818	0.228107112
ENSG00000206559	ZCWPW2	0.929444	0.031776955	0.038502406
ENSG00000197114	ZGPAT	0.890333	0.050447624	0.09943705
ENSG00000165156	ZHX1	0.999495	0.000219258	0.427467343
ENSG00000121741	ZMYM2	0.82584	0.083104152	0.270994479
ENSG00000015171	ZMYND11	0.959348	0.018023904	0.235639846
ENSG00000101040	ZMYND8	0.94716	0.023576596	0.292339038
ENSG00000121988	ZRANB3	0.926406	0.033198634	0.159745896
ENSG00000036549	ZZZ3	0.996246	0.001633385	0.14347317

2.9.3 Additional file 3: Table S2: Expression of BRDT in ESCC.

sample	samples	histological_type	*BRDT* expression
TCGA-LN-A49Y-01	TCGA-LN-A49Y-01	Esophagus Squamous Cell Carcinoma	10.41
TCGA-JY-A6FD-01	TCGA-JY-A6FD-01	Esophagus Squamous Cell Carcinoma	9.522
TCGA-XP-A8T6-01	TCGA-XP-A8T6-01	Esophagus Squamous Cell Carcinoma	9.245
TCGA-LN-A7HY-01	TCGA-LN-A7HY-01	Esophagus Squamous Cell Carcinoma	9.135
TCGA-Z6-A8JD-01	TCGA-Z6-A8JD-01	Esophagus Squamous Cell Carcinoma	8.493
TCGA-IG-A5B8-01	TCGA-IG-A5B8-01	Esophagus Squamous Cell Carcinoma	8.44
TCGA-VR-A8Q7-01	TCGA-VR-A8Q7-01	Esophagus Squamous Cell Carcinoma	8.426
TCGA-VR-A8EP-01	TCGA-VR-A8EP-01	Esophagus Squamous Cell Carcinoma	8.035
TCGA-LN-A49S-01	TCGA-LN-A49S-01	Esophagus Squamous Cell Carcinoma	7.805
TCGA-LN-A49W-01	TCGA-LN-A49W-01	Esophagus Squamous Cell Carcinoma	7.785
TCGA-LN-A4A4-01	TCGA-LN-A4A4-01	Esophagus Squamous Cell Carcinoma	7.405
TCGA-IG-A51D-01	TCGA-IG-A51D-01	Esophagus Squamous Cell Carcinoma	7.403
TCGA-IG-A3QL-01	TCGA-IG-A3QL-01	Esophagus Squamous Cell Carcinoma	7.212
TCGA-LN-A4A6-01	TCGA-LN-A4A6-01	Esophagus Squamous Cell Carcinoma	7.138
TCGA-LN-A9FP-01	TCGA-LN-A9FP-01	Esophagus Squamous Cell Carcinoma	6.921
TCGA-L7-A56G-01	TCGA-L7-A56G-01	Esophagus Squamous Cell Carcinoma	6.901
TCGA-LN-A4A3-01	TCGA-LN-A4A3-01	Esophagus Squamous Cell Carcinoma	6.346
TCGA-LN-A49N-01	TCGA-LN-A49N-01	Esophagus Squamous Cell Carcinoma	5.943
TCGA-LN-A4A8-01	TCGA-LN-A4A8-01	Esophagus Squamous Cell Carcinoma	5.399
TCGA-LN-A9FO-01	TCGA-LN-A9FO-01	Esophagus Squamous Cell Carcinoma	5.307
TCGA-LN-A4A5-01	TCGA-LN-A4A5-01	Esophagus Squamous Cell Carcinoma	4.437
TCGA-LN-A49P-01	TCGA-LN-A49P-01	Esophagus Squamous Cell Carcinoma	3.711
TCGA-IG-A50L-01	TCGA-IG-A50L-01	Esophagus Squamous Cell Carcinoma	3.484
TCGA-IG-A97H-01	TCGA-IG-A97H-01	Esophagus Squamous Cell Carcinoma	3.404

TCGA-VR-A8EX-01	TCGA-VR-A8EX-01	Esophagus Squamous Cell Carcinoma	2.645
TCGA-IG-A4P3-01	TCGA-IG-A4P3-01	Esophagus Squamous Cell Carcinoma	2.483
TCGA-IG-A4QT-01	TCGA-IG-A4QT-01	Esophagus Squamous Cell Carcinoma	1.998
TCGA-VR-A8ET-01	TCGA-VR-A8ET-01	Esophagus Squamous Cell Carcinoma	1.734
TCGA-L5-A88S-01	TCGA-L5-A88S-01	Esophagus Squamous Cell Carcinoma	1.437
TCGA-VR-A8EO-01	TCGA-VR-A8EO-01	Esophagus Squamous Cell Carcinoma	1.389
TCGA-IG-A3YC-01	TCGA-IG-A3YC-01	Esophagus Squamous Cell Carcinoma	1.128
TCGA-Z6-A8JE-01	TCGA-Z6-A8JE-01	Esophagus Squamous Cell Carcinoma	1.089
TCGA-LN-A4A9-01	TCGA-LN-A4A9-01	Esophagus Squamous Cell Carcinoma	1.036
TCGA-LN-A4A2-01	TCGA-LN-A4A2-01	Esophagus Squamous Cell Carcinoma	0.7973
TCGA-IG-A3I8-11	TCGA-IG-A3I8-11	Esophagus Squamous Cell Carcinoma	0.6947
TCGA-L5-A4OM-01	TCGA-L5-A4OM-01	Esophagus Squamous Cell Carcinoma	0.6836
TCGA-VR-AA7B-01	TCGA-VR-AA7B-01	Esophagus Squamous Cell Carcinoma	0.6043
TCGA-IG-A3YA-01	TCGA-IG-A3YA-01	Esophagus Squamous Cell Carcinoma	0.5832
TCGA-VR-AA7D-01	TCGA-VR-AA7D-01	Esophagus Squamous Cell Carcinoma	0.5575
TCGA-LN-A49L-01	TCGA-LN-A49L-01	Esophagus Squamous Cell Carcinoma	0.5378
TCGA-LN-A8I0-01	TCGA-LN-A8I0-01	Esophagus Squamous Cell Carcinoma	0.4936
TCGA-VR-A8ER-01	TCGA-VR-A8ER-01	Esophagus Squamous Cell Carcinoma	0.4674
TCGA-LN-A4MQ-01	TCGA-LN-A4MQ-01	Esophagus Squamous Cell Carcinoma	0.4532
TCGA-Z6-A9VB-01	TCGA-Z6-A9VB-01	Esophagus Squamous Cell Carcinoma	0.4162
TCGA-LN-A9FQ-01	TCGA-LN-A9FQ-01	Esophagus Squamous Cell Carcinoma	0.412
TCGA-VR-AA4G-01	TCGA-VR-AA4G-01	Esophagus Squamous Cell Carcinoma	0.4082
TCGA-LN-A5U5-01	TCGA-LN-A5U5-01	Esophagus Squamous Cell Carcinoma	0.4069
TCGA-V5-A7RC-01	TCGA-V5-A7RC-01	Esophagus Squamous Cell Carcinoma	0.4003
TCGA-L5-A88Z-01	TCGA-L5-A88Z-01	Esophagus Squamous Cell Carcinoma	0.3942
TCGA-IG-A97I-01	TCGA-IG-A97I-01	Esophagus Squamous Cell Carcinoma	0.379
TCGA-IG-A8O2-01	TCGA-IG-A8O2-01	Esophagus Squamous Cell Carcinoma	0.3757

TCGA-Q9-A6FU-01	TCGA-Q9-A6FU-01	Esophagus Squamous Cell Carcinoma	0.2711
TCGA-IC-A6RF-01	TCGA-IC-A6RF-01	Esophagus Squamous Cell Carcinoma	0
TCGA-IC-A6RF-11	TCGA-IC-A6RF-11	Esophagus Squamous Cell Carcinoma	0
TCGA-IG-A3I8-01	TCGA-IG-A3I8-01	Esophagus Squamous Cell Carcinoma	0
TCGA-IG-A3Y9-01	TCGA-IG-A3Y9-01	Esophagus Squamous Cell Carcinoma	0
TCGA-IG-A3YB-01	TCGA-IG-A3YB-01	Esophagus Squamous Cell Carcinoma	0
TCGA-IG-A5S3-01	TCGA-IG-A5S3-01	Esophagus Squamous Cell Carcinoma	0
TCGA-IG-A625-01	TCGA-IG-A625-01	Esophagus Squamous Cell Carcinoma	0
TCGA-IG-A6QS-01	TCGA-IG-A6QS-01	Esophagus Squamous Cell Carcinoma	0
TCGA-JY-A6FA-01	TCGA-JY-A6FA-01	Esophagus Squamous Cell Carcinoma	0
TCGA-JY-A6FE-01	TCGA-JY-A6FE-01	Esophagus Squamous Cell Carcinoma	0
TCGA-JY-A6FG-01	TCGA-JY-A6FG-01	Esophagus Squamous Cell Carcinoma	0
TCGA-JY-A93F-01	TCGA-JY-A93F-01	Esophagus Squamous Cell Carcinoma	0
TCGA-KH-A6WC-01	TCGA-KH-A6WC-01	Esophagus Squamous Cell Carcinoma	0
TCGA-L5-A43H-01	TCGA-L5-A43H-01	Esophagus Squamous Cell Carcinoma	0
TCGA-L5-A43J-01	TCGA-L5-A43J-01	Esophagus Squamous Cell Carcinoma	0
TCGA-L5-A4OM-11	TCGA-L5-A4OM-11	Esophagus Squamous Cell Carcinoma	0
TCGA-L5-A88W-01	TCGA-L5-A88W-01	Esophagus Squamous Cell Carcinoma	0
TCGA-L5-A8NK-01	TCGA-L5-A8NK-01	Esophagus Squamous Cell Carcinoma	0
TCGA-L5-A8NQ-01	TCGA-L5-A8NQ-01	Esophagus Squamous Cell Carcinoma	0
TCGA-LN-A49K-01	TCGA-LN-A49K-01	Esophagus Squamous Cell Carcinoma	0
TCGA-LN-A49M-01	TCGA-LN-A49M-01	Esophagus Squamous Cell Carcinoma	0
TCGA-LN-A49O-01	TCGA-LN-A49O-01	Esophagus Squamous Cell Carcinoma	0
TCGA-LN-A49R-01	TCGA-LN-A49R-01	Esophagus Squamous Cell Carcinoma	0
TCGA-LN-A49U-01	TCGA-LN-A49U-01	Esophagus Squamous Cell Carcinoma	0
TCGA-LN-A49V-01	TCGA-LN-A49V-01	Esophagus Squamous Cell Carcinoma	0
TCGA-LN-A49X-01	TCGA-LN-A49X-01	Esophagus Squamous Cell Carcinoma	0

TCGA-LN-A4A1-01	TCGA-LN-A4A1-01	Esophagus Squamous Cell Carcinoma	0
TCGA-LN-A4MR-01	TCGA-LN-A4MR-01	Esophagus Squamous Cell Carcinoma	0
TCGA-LN-A5U6-01	TCGA-LN-A5U6-01	Esophagus Squamous Cell Carcinoma	0
TCGA-LN-A5U7-01	TCGA-LN-A5U7-01	Esophagus Squamous Cell Carcinoma	0
TCGA-LN-A7HV-01	TCGA-LN-A7HV-01	Esophagus Squamous Cell Carcinoma	0
TCGA-LN-A7HW-01	TCGA-LN-A7HW-01	Esophagus Squamous Cell Carcinoma	0
TCGA-LN-A7HX-01	TCGA-LN-A7HX-01	Esophagus Squamous Cell Carcinoma	0
TCGA-LN-A7HZ-01	TCGA-LN-A7HZ-01	Esophagus Squamous Cell Carcinoma	0
TCGA-LN-A8HZ-01	TCGA-LN-A8HZ-01	Esophagus Squamous Cell Carcinoma	0
TCGA-LN-A8I1-01	TCGA-LN-A8I1-01	Esophagus Squamous Cell Carcinoma	0
TCGA-LN-A9FR-01	TCGA-LN-A9FR-01	Esophagus Squamous Cell Carcinoma	0
TCGA-S8-A6BW-01	TCGA-S8-A6BW-01	Esophagus Squamous Cell Carcinoma	0
TCGA-V5-A7RC-06	TCGA-V5-A7RC-06	Esophagus Squamous Cell Carcinoma	0
TCGA-V5-AASV-01	TCGA-V5-AASV-01	Esophagus Squamous Cell Carcinoma	0
TCGA-VR-A8EU-01	TCGA-VR-A8EU-01	Esophagus Squamous Cell Carcinoma	0
TCGA-VR-A8EW-01	TCGA-VR-A8EW-01	Esophagus Squamous Cell Carcinoma	0
TCGA-VR-A8EY-01	TCGA-VR-A8EY-01	Esophagus Squamous Cell Carcinoma	0
TCGA-VR-A8EZ-01	TCGA-VR-A8EZ-01	Esophagus Squamous Cell Carcinoma	0
TCGA-VR-AA7I-01	TCGA-VR-AA7I-01	Esophagus Squamous Cell Carcinoma	0
TCGA-XP-A8T8-01	TCGA-XP-A8T8-01	Esophagus Squamous Cell Carcinoma	0
TCGA-Z6-AAPN-01	TCGA-Z6-AAPN-01	Esophagus Squamous Cell Carcinoma	0
TCGA-XP-A8T7-01	TCGA-XP-A8T7-01	Esophagus Squamous Cell Carcinoma	NA
TCGA-L5-A4OF-01	TCGA-L5-A4OF-01	Esophagus Adenocarcinoma, NOS	8.66
TCGA-2H-A9GQ-01	TCGA-2H-A9GQ-01	Esophagus Adenocarcinoma, NOS	8.231
TCGA-2H-A9GO-01	TCGA-2H-A9GO-01	Esophagus Adenocarcinoma, NOS	6.833
TCGA-JY-A93D-01	TCGA-JY-A93D-01	Esophagus Adenocarcinoma, NOS	4.387
TCGA-2H-A9GF-01	TCGA-2H-A9GF-01	Esophagus Adenocarcinoma, NOS	3.595

TCGA-VR-A8EQ-01	TCGA-VR-A8EQ-01	Esophagus Adenocarcinoma, NOS	3.169
TCGA-R6-A6XG-01	TCGA-R6-A6XG-01	Esophagus Adenocarcinoma, NOS	2.994
TCGA-L5-A4OG-11	TCGA-L5-A4OG-11	Esophagus Adenocarcinoma, NOS	2.56
TCGA-L5-A891-01	TCGA-L5-A891-01	Esophagus Adenocarcinoma, NOS	2.529
TCGA-JY-A6FB-01	TCGA-JY-A6FB-01	Esophagus Adenocarcinoma, NOS	2.479
TCGA-L5-A4OO-11	TCGA-L5-A4OO-11	Esophagus Adenocarcinoma, NOS	2.366
TCGA-L5-A8NL-01	TCGA-L5-A8NL-01	Esophagus Adenocarcinoma, NOS	2.208
TCGA-2H-A9GL-01	TCGA-2H-A9GL-01	Esophagus Adenocarcinoma, NOS	1.795
TCGA-L5-A4OW-01	TCGA-L5-A4OW-01	Esophagus Adenocarcinoma, NOS	1.535
TCGA-L5-A8NR-01	TCGA-L5-A8NR-01	Esophagus Adenocarcinoma, NOS	1.425
TCGA-L5-A893-01	TCGA-L5-A893-01	Esophagus Adenocarcinoma, NOS	1.401
TCGA-L5-A8NU-01	TCGA-L5-A8NU-01	Esophagus Adenocarcinoma, NOS	1.345
TCGA-R6-A6KZ-01	TCGA-R6-A6KZ-01	Esophagus Adenocarcinoma, NOS	1.289
TCGA-2H-A9GK-01	TCGA-2H-A9GK-01	Esophagus Adenocarcinoma, NOS	1.203
TCGA-L7-A6VZ-01	TCGA-L7-A6VZ-01	Esophagus Adenocarcinoma, NOS	1.194
TCGA-ZR-A9CJ-01	TCGA-ZR-A9CJ-01	Esophagus Adenocarcinoma, NOS	1.106
TCGA-R6-A6XQ-01	TCGA-R6-A6XQ-01	Esophagus Adenocarcinoma, NOS	0.942
TCGA-R6-A6DQ-01	TCGA-R6-A6DQ-01	Esophagus Adenocarcinoma, NOS	0.931
TCGA-V5-A7RB-01	TCGA-V5-A7RB-01	Esophagus Adenocarcinoma, NOS	0.9195
TCGA-L5-A8NG-01	TCGA-L5-A8NG-01	Esophagus Adenocarcinoma, NOS	0.7806
TCGA-L5-A4OF-11	TCGA-L5-A4OF-11	Esophagus Adenocarcinoma, NOS	0.7202
TCGA-Q9-A6FW-01	TCGA-Q9-A6FW-01	Esophagus Adenocarcinoma, NOS	0.7088
TCGA-IC-A6RE-11	TCGA-IC-A6RE-11	Esophagus Adenocarcinoma, NOS	0.6895
TCGA-2H-A9GJ-01	TCGA-2H-A9GJ-01	Esophagus Adenocarcinoma, NOS	0.6869
TCGA-L5-A4OJ-01	TCGA-L5-A4OJ-01	Esophagus Adenocarcinoma, NOS	0.6621
TCGA-R6-A6L4-01	TCGA-R6-A6L4-01	Esophagus Adenocarcinoma, NOS	0.5745
TCGA-L5-A4OU-01	TCGA-L5-A4OU-01	Esophagus Adenocarcinoma, NOS	0.5351

TCGA-JY-A938-01	TCGA-JY-A938-01	Esophagus Adenocarcinoma, NOS	0.4502
TCGA-X8-AAAR-01	TCGA-X8-AAAR-01	Esophagus Adenocarcinoma, NOS	0.4263
TCGA-L5-A43M-01	TCGA-L5-A43M-01	Esophagus Adenocarcinoma, NOS	0.3807
TCGA-JY-A93C-01	TCGA-JY-A93C-01	Esophagus Adenocarcinoma, NOS	0.3797
TCGA-V5-A7RE-01	TCGA-V5-A7RE-01	Esophagus Adenocarcinoma, NOS	0.3717
TCGA-L5-A4OE-01	TCGA-L5-A4OE-01	Esophagus Adenocarcinoma, NOS	0.3533
TCGA-L5-A8NI-01	TCGA-L5-A8NI-01	Esophagus Adenocarcinoma, NOS	0.3497
TCGA-L5-A4OX-01	TCGA-L5-A4OX-01	Esophagus Adenocarcinoma, NOS	0.3415
TCGA-R6-A6Y2-01	TCGA-R6-A6Y2-01	Esophagus Adenocarcinoma, NOS	0.3193
TCGA-L5-A4OQ-01	TCGA-L5-A4OQ-01	Esophagus Adenocarcinoma, NOS	0.2855
TCGA-L5-A4OR-01	TCGA-L5-A4OR-01	Esophagus Adenocarcinoma, NOS	0.2754
TCGA-2H-A9GG-01	TCGA-2H-A9GG-01	Esophagus Adenocarcinoma, NOS	0
TCGA-2H-A9GH-01	TCGA-2H-A9GH-01	Esophagus Adenocarcinoma, NOS	0
TCGA-2H-A9GI-01	TCGA-2H-A9GI-01	Esophagus Adenocarcinoma, NOS	0
TCGA-2H-A9GM-01	TCGA-2H-A9GM-01	Esophagus Adenocarcinoma, NOS	0
TCGA-2H-A9GN-01	TCGA-2H-A9GN-01	Esophagus Adenocarcinoma, NOS	0
TCGA-2H-A9GR-01	TCGA-2H-A9GR-01	Esophagus Adenocarcinoma, NOS	0
TCGA-IC-A6RE-01	TCGA-IC-A6RE-01	Esophagus Adenocarcinoma, NOS	0
TCGA-IG-A4QS-01	TCGA-IG-A4QS-01	Esophagus Adenocarcinoma, NOS	0
TCGA-IG-A7DP-01	TCGA-IG-A7DP-01	Esophagus Adenocarcinoma, NOS	0
TCGA-JY-A6F8-01	TCGA-JY-A6F8-01	Esophagus Adenocarcinoma, NOS	0
TCGA-JY-A6FH-01	TCGA-JY-A6FH-01	Esophagus Adenocarcinoma, NOS	0
TCGA-JY-A939-01	TCGA-JY-A939-01	Esophagus Adenocarcinoma, NOS	0
TCGA-JY-A93E-01	TCGA-JY-A93E-01	Esophagus Adenocarcinoma, NOS	0
TCGA-L5-A43C-01	TCGA-L5-A43C-01	Esophagus Adenocarcinoma, NOS	0
TCGA-L5-A43C-11	TCGA-L5-A43C-11	Esophagus Adenocarcinoma, NOS	0
TCGA-L5-A43E-01	TCGA-L5-A43E-01	Esophagus Adenocarcinoma, NOS	0

TCGA-L5-A43I-01	TCGA-L5-A43I-01	Esophagus Adenocarcinoma, NOS	0
TCGA-L5-A4OG-01	TCGA-L5-A4OG-01	Esophagus Adenocarcinoma, NOS	0
TCGA-L5-A4OH-01	TCGA-L5-A4OH-01	Esophagus Adenocarcinoma, NOS	0
TCGA-L5-A4OI-01	TCGA-L5-A4OI-01	Esophagus Adenocarcinoma, NOS	0
TCGA-L5-A4OJ-11	TCGA-L5-A4OJ-11	Esophagus Adenocarcinoma, NOS	0
TCGA-L5-A4ON-01	TCGA-L5-A4ON-01	Esophagus Adenocarcinoma, NOS	0
TCGA-L5-A4OO-01	TCGA-L5-A4OO-01	Esophagus Adenocarcinoma, NOS	0
TCGA-L5-A4OP-01	TCGA-L5-A4OP-01	Esophagus Adenocarcinoma, NOS	0
TCGA-L5-A4OQ-11	TCGA-L5-A4OQ-11	Esophagus Adenocarcinoma, NOS	0
TCGA-L5-A4OR-11	TCGA-L5-A4OR-11	Esophagus Adenocarcinoma, NOS	0
TCGA-L5-A4OS-01	TCGA-L5-A4OS-01	Esophagus Adenocarcinoma, NOS	0
TCGA-L5-A4OT-01	TCGA-L5-A4OT-01	Esophagus Adenocarcinoma, NOS	0
TCGA-L5-A88T-01	TCGA-L5-A88T-01	Esophagus Adenocarcinoma, NOS	0
TCGA-L5-A88V-01	TCGA-L5-A88V-01	Esophagus Adenocarcinoma, NOS	0
TCGA-L5-A88Y-01	TCGA-L5-A88Y-01	Esophagus Adenocarcinoma, NOS	0
TCGA-L5-A8NE-01	TCGA-L5-A8NE-01	Esophagus Adenocarcinoma, NOS	0
TCGA-L5-A8NF-01	TCGA-L5-A8NF-01	Esophagus Adenocarcinoma, NOS	0
TCGA-L5-A8NH-01	TCGA-L5-A8NH-01	Esophagus Adenocarcinoma, NOS	0
TCGA-L5-A8NJ-01	TCGA-L5-A8NJ-01	Esophagus Adenocarcinoma, NOS	0
TCGA-L5-A8NM-01	TCGA-L5-A8NM-01	Esophagus Adenocarcinoma, NOS	0
TCGA-L5-A8NN-01	TCGA-L5-A8NN-01	Esophagus Adenocarcinoma, NOS	0
TCGA-L5-A8NS-01	TCGA-L5-A8NS-01	Esophagus Adenocarcinoma, NOS	0
TCGA-L5-A8NT-01	TCGA-L5-A8NT-01	Esophagus Adenocarcinoma, NOS	0
TCGA-L5-A8NV-01	TCGA-L5-A8NV-01	Esophagus Adenocarcinoma, NOS	0
TCGA-L5-A8NW-01	TCGA-L5-A8NW-01	Esophagus Adenocarcinoma, NOS	0
TCGA-M9-A5M8-01	TCGA-M9-A5M8-01	Esophagus Adenocarcinoma, NOS	0
TCGA-R6-A6DN-01	TCGA-R6-A6DN-01	Esophagus Adenocarcinoma, NOS	0

TCGA-R6-A6L6-01	TCGA-R6-A6L6-01	Esophagus Adenocarcinoma, NOS	0
TCGA-R6-A6Y0-01	TCGA-R6-A6Y0-01	Esophagus Adenocarcinoma, NOS	0
TCGA-R6-A8W5-01	TCGA-R6-A8W5-01	Esophagus Adenocarcinoma, NOS	0
TCGA-R6-A8W8-01	TCGA-R6-A8W8-01	Esophagus Adenocarcinoma, NOS	0
TCGA-R6-A8WC-01	TCGA-R6-A8WC-01	Esophagus Adenocarcinoma, NOS	0
TCGA-R6-A8WG-01	TCGA-R6-A8WG-01	Esophagus Adenocarcinoma, NOS	0
TCGA-RE-A7BO-01	TCGA-RE-A7BO-01	Esophagus Adenocarcinoma, NOS	0
TCGA-S8-A6BV-01	TCGA-S8-A6BV-01	Esophagus Adenocarcinoma, NOS	0
TCGA-V5-AASW-01	TCGA-V5-AASW-01	Esophagus Adenocarcinoma, NOS	0
TCGA-V5-AASX-01	TCGA-V5-AASX-01	Esophagus Adenocarcinoma, NOS	0
TCGA-VR-AA4D-01	TCGA-VR-AA4D-01	Esophagus Adenocarcinoma, NOS	0
TCGA-L5-A4OE-11	TCGA-L5-A4OE-11	Esophagus Adenocarcinoma, NOS	NA
TCGA-L5-A4OH-11	TCGA-L5-A4OH-11	Esophagus Adenocarcinoma, NOS	NA
TCGA-L5-A4OI-11	TCGA-L5-A4OI-11	Esophagus Adenocarcinoma, NOS	NA
TCGA-L5-A4ON-11	TCGA-L5-A4ON-11	Esophagus Adenocarcinoma, NOS	NA
TCGA-L5-A4OP-11	TCGA-L5-A4OP-11	Esophagus Adenocarcinoma, NOS	NA
TCGA-V5-A7RE-11	TCGA-V5-A7RE-11	Esophagus Adenocarcinoma, NOS	NA
TCGA-V5-AASX-11	TCGA-V5-AASX-11	Esophagus Adenocarcinoma, NOS	NA

2.9.4 Additional file 4: Table S3: siRNAs used in this study.

Name	Sequence (5' to 3')
Non-targeting siRNA #5	UGGUUUACAUGUCGACUAA
BRDT #2	CAAAUCAACUUCAGUAUCU
BRDT #3	GAAAAUGGAUAACCAAGAA
BRDT #4	GUAGAGAGAACACUAAUGA
BRDT #18	GAGAUAAACUUGGGCGAGU
TP63 #5	CAUCAUGUCUGGACUAUUU
TP63 #8	CGACAGUCUUGUACAAUUU
FAT2	Smart pool, Cat. NO: M-011270-00-0005

2.9.5 Additional file 5: Table S4: Primers used in this study (5'-3').

Name	Forward	Reverse	Purposes
GPADH	ATGGGGAAGGTGAAGGTCG	GGGGTCATTGATGGCAACAATA	Gene expression
BRDT	GAGTCTGAAAGTAGCAGCAGTGA	TATCCTATCTGTGTGACGCCTGT	Gene expression
FAT2	GCCACACAGGTCCACATCTT	GATCTATGGCCTGGACTCGC	Gene expression
KRT14	CAGAGATGTGACCTCCTCCA	CTCAGTTCTTGGTGCGAAGG	Gene expression
PTHLH	AGCCGCCGCCTCAAAAG	AGCTGTGTGGATTTCTGCGA	Gene expression
TP63	TTTAGTGAGCCACAGTACACGAA	GAGAGCATCGAAGGTGGAGC	Gene expression
hnFAT2	CCCACCCCCAGTACCTGTAT	AGGACGATGACAGTGGCTTG	Gene expression
hnKRT14	CCATTCACCCACCTTGTTCCT	CCGACCTGGAAGTGAAGATCC	Gene expression
hnPTHLH	GATGGGGCACTTACAGGCG	GAGACTGGTTCAGCAGTGGAG	Gene expression
BRDT-Ex5 (Osaka)	ATCACCCAGCGCAACAGAAA	CCTTTTGTAACTTGGGCCGC	Gene expression
ACTB (Osaka)	CGCTCTCTGCTCCTCCTGTTC	ATCCGTTGACTCCGACCTTCAC	Gene expression
BRDT	CATTCTGTGAGAACAGGGCA	ACCCAAACAGTACAAATTCTACCTA	Genotyping
BRDT-gRNA-1	ATTCTGGCTCATACTTTTCC	NA	Genome editing
BRDT-gRNA-2	TTTATGAATAGACACCTAAG	NA	Genome editing

2.9.6 Additional file 6: Table S5: Antibodies used in this study.

Target	Purpose	Quantity	Source	Catalog
BRDT	WB, ChIP	1:1000, 10 µL	Cell signaling	#65133
BRDT	IP	6 µg	Santa Cruz	sc-515674
IgG	IP	6 µg	Diagenode	C15410206
p63	WB, ChIP	1:1000, 2 µg	Santa Cruz	sc-8431
H3K27ac	ChIP	1 µg	Diagenode	C15410196
H3K9ac	ChIP	1 µg	Diagenode	C15410004
H4K5ac	ChIP	1 µg	Diagenode	C15410025
H3K4me1	ChIP	1 µg	Diagenode	C15410194
H3K4me3	ChIP	1 µg	Diagenode	C15410003
H3K27me3	ChIP	1 µg	Diagenode	C15410069
BRD2	WB	1:1000	Cell signaling	#5848
BRD3	WB	1:1000	Bethyl	A302-368
BRD4	WB	1:1000	Diagenode	C15410337
GAPDH	WB	1:5000	Origene	TA802519

CHAPTER 3: General discussion

ESCC, the predominant subtype of esophageal cancer, is a deadly malignancy with a poor 5-year survival rate of 15 to 20% (Siegel et al., 2019). Currently, there is no effective therapy available and many clinical trials targeting the EGFR signaling pathway have not yielded any encouraging results, highlighting the necessity for identifying novel therapeutic targets. Recent genomic studies showed that many epigenetic factors, such as p300 and KMT2D, are also mutated, suggesting an epigenetic dysregulation in ESCC (Gao et al., 2014; Kim et al., 2017; Lin et al., 2014; Sawada et al., 2016; Song et al., 2014). Given the lack of therapeutic targets and the importance of epigenetic factors, we decided to systematically screen epigenetic factors for potential therapeutic targets. First of all, we designed an unbiased screening comprising two aspects: tissue specificity in normal tissues and differential expression among ESCC patients. We then identified BRDT, the bromodomains-testis specific protein, as a novel target. Subsequently, we validated the aberrant expression of *BRDT* in ESCC using an independent cohort. Because BRDT is a testis-specific protein, all studies investing the function of BRDT were carried out in the context of germ cells (Gaucher et al., 2012; Pivot-Pajot et al., 2003) and the role (if there is) of BRDT in the field of cancer biology has yet to be explored. Experimental studies in ESCC cell lines showed that BRDT does not affect cell proliferation but is indispensable for cell migration. Transcriptomic profiling (RNA-seq) following the depletion of BRDT revealed that BRDT regulates many ECM-related pathways, which can explain the loss of cell migratory potential. After that, genome occupancy profiling (ChIP-seq) uncovered that BRDT is preferentially localized at promoters and enhancers. Moreover, the binding motif of ΔNp63, a squamous-lineage determinant (Mills et al., 1999; Yang et al., 1999), was found in BRDT-bound region, indicating the co-localization of BRDT and ΔNp63. We then found that BRDT can regulate a subset of p63 targets, such as *FAT2*, *KRT14* and *PTHLH*. In order to understand the mechanism underlying BRDT controlling the expression ΔNp63 targets, we combined epigenome and chromatin long-range interaction data and found that BRDT co-localizes with ΔNp63 at certain super enhancers which can loop back to their target genes. Finally, we could duplicate the effects caused by the loss of BRDT on gene expression by pharmacologically depleting BRDT using MZ1, a PROTAC compound targeting BET proteins. A hypothetical model of BRDT regulating p63 target gene expression via super enhancers is shown in Fig. 22. Taken together, these results established the functional role of BRDT in ESCC and provided a potential therapeutic target for precision medicine.

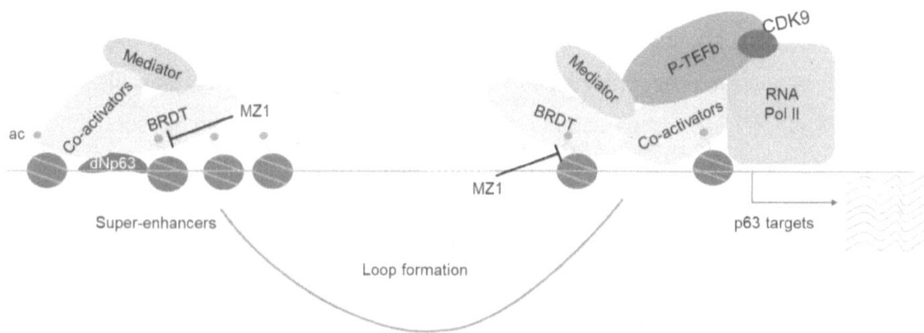

Fig. 22 A hypothetical model of BRDT regulating p63 target genes. ΔNp63 binds to the super enhancer site and recruits transcription co-activators which can modify histones and affect chromatin accessibility. BRDT is also recruited to the super enhancer site, leading to the further activation of the super enhancer. Through looping the complex formed at the super enhancer is brought in close proximity to its target gene, promoting gene transcription. This process can be disrupted by MZ1, a PROTAC compound targeting BET proteins.

3.1 BRDT: A cancer/testis antigen

Under normal physiological conditions, BRDT is only expressed in the testes, but it can be aberrantly expressed in several cancer entities, such as lung, breast, head and neck, and esophageal cancer. This is not a novel phenomenon and the identification of the aberrant expression of testes-specific genes dates back to the 1990s (Traversari et al., 1992), when MAGEA1 (Melanoma-Associated Antigen A1) was identified during autologous typing. Since then, a growing number of genes with a cancer/testis-restricted expression pattern was identified and prompted people to categorize them as a family (Chen et al., 1997). They were named cancer/testis antigens (CTAs) because of their restricted expression and MAGEA1 became the founding member. Two decades ago, the expression of *BRDT* was detected in lung cancer along with other CTAs, such as MAGEA1, MAGEC1 (Melanoma-Associated Antigen C1), MAGEC2 (Melanoma-Associated Antigen C2), SSX4 (SSX Family Member 4) and NY-ESO1 (New York Esophageal Squamous Cell Carcinoma-1) (Scanlan et al., 2000). The expression of these CTAs in a significant subgroup of patients revealed the aberrant activation of the gametogenic program in cancer cells which has led to a theory that the gametogenic program is one of the driving forces of carcinogenesis (Simpson et al., 2005). This theory is supported by many reports showing the role of CTAs in cell proliferation, migration and invasion (Doyle et al., 2010; Liu et al., 2008a; Maine et al., 2016). Additionally, CTAs, such as MAGE family proteins, also confer resistance to chemotherapeutic agents (Monte et al., 2006). We also tested whether BRDT confers any chemoresistance, but no correlation between the expression of BRDT and chemo-responsiveness was found (Supplemental Fig. S4). Interestingly, CTCFL (CCCTC-Binding Factor Like), another potential target from our screening (Fig. 16A), has also been reported to have an oncogenic role (Renaud et al., 2011; Zampieri et al., 2014). Its specific role in ESCC remains to be explored. Collectively, our data also suggests that BRDT, a CTA, cooperates with ΔNp63 to enhance ESCC cell migration, thus displaying an oncogenic function in ESCC.

3.2 BRDT and chromatin remodeling

Spermatogenesis involves a genome-wide chromatin remodeling, more specifically chromatin compaction mediated by histone-to-protamine transition (Rathke et al., 2014). Interestingly, in previous studies, the ectopic expression of Brdt was not able to induce chromatin compaction unless the cells were pre-treated with TSA, an HDAC inhibitor. This suggests that the induction of chromatin compaction is dependent on the hyper acetylation of the genome, which is, in turn, recognized by BD-containing proteins (Gaucher et al., 2012). In another study, Brdt-immunoprecipitation followed by mass spectrometry (MS) was exploited to examine the interactome of Brdt (Dhar et al., 2012). Top candidates interacting with Brdt included Top1 (DNA Topoisomerase 1) and Smarce1, a subunit of the SWI/SNF chromatin remodeling complex (Fig. 23). The N-terminal region of Brdt is responsible for recognizing acetylated histones and interacting with Smarce1, indicating the interaction with Smarce1 is mediated by histone acetylation. Indeed, hyperacetylation of histone can enhance the interaction between Brdt and Smarce1, confirming that the Brdt-Smarce1 interaction is acetylation-dependent (Dhar et al., 2012). Another study showed that exogenously expressed BRDT interacts with HDAC1, PRMT5 (Protein Arginine Methyltransferase 5) and TRIM28, which can potentially influence the chromatin state as well (Wang and Wolgemuth, 2016). Thus, BRDT interacts with several factors involved in chromatin remodeling and could therefore influence chromatin accesibility in the cell, although the exact mechanism by which BRDT induces such changes remains elusive.

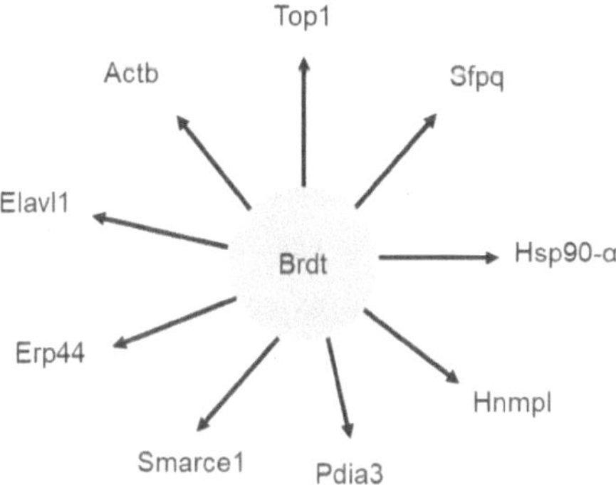

Fig. 23 Top Brdt-interacting partners in rat testes. (Dhar et al., 2012)

Given the importance of chromatin accessibility in gene expression, we expected that the ectopic expression of BRDT would lead to massive chromatin rearrangement upon HDAC inhibition, potentially leading to altered gene expression which may affect multiple cellular processes. A naïve guess was that cell proliferation could be affected, so we hypothesized that the ectopic expression of BRDT increases the sensitivity of ESCCs to HDAC inhibition. However, a preliminary proliferation study did not seem to stand in line with the expectation: the depletion of BRDT does not seem to alter the responsiveness to the tested HDAC inhibitors: Mocetinostat and Vorinostat (Supplemental Fig. S5). There are a few possible explanations: 1. Proliferation might not be the best readout for assessing the alteration of gene expression following the hyperacetylation-mediated chromatin remodeling; 2. BRDT may have a completely different interactome (e.g. ΔNp63 instead of SMARCE1) in ESCC cell lines compared to germ cells leading a shift of its biological function; 3. BRDT-induced chromatin remodeling could happen in a much smaller scale due to the different cellular context and proliferation-related genes might not be directly affected by these potential localized chromatin remodeling events.

In our cell system, BRDT affects cell migration and this may or may not be mediated by chromatin remodeling. To answer this, we can test examine the migratory potential of cells upon the depletion of BRDT and HDAC inhibition. Furthermore, the interactome of BRDT may be different in ESCC compared to germ cells, as we did not observe that BRDT interacts with the previously described interacting partners (Fig. 23). In fact, in ESCC we show that the binding specificity of BRDT could be determined by its interacting partners, such as ΔNp63. Therefore, interactome data in ESCC would be helpful to systematically characterize the role of BRDT in cancer and more specifically in esophageal cancer. Finally, to reveal the effect of BRDT on chromatin organization, we can perform a HiC experiment upon BRDT-loss and analyze if there is any change in chromatin conformation. In this project, we conducted an H3K27ac HiChIP in control and BRDT-KD cells. Unfortunately, due to technical issues, the quality of our data was not good enough to provide any quantitative result. Therefore, the role of BRDT in chromatin organization remains to be explored.

3.3 BRDT vs BRD4: Differences and similarities

BRDT and BRD4 are closely related to each other because of their high degree of sequence similarity. Among the BET family members, only BRD4 and BRDT possess a CTD, a domain involved in positive regulation of transcription elongation through interaction with P-TEFb (Gaucher et al., 2012; Moon et al., 2005; Yang et al., 2005). Because of the sequence similarity, especially in the CTD (Bisgrove et al., 2007), BRDT is also referred to as the testis-specific paralog of BRD4 (Gaucher et al., 2012). Given the importance of BRD4 and BRDT in transcription regulation, it is not surprising that the depletion of them would lead to the downregulation of a large number of genes (Gaucher et al., 2012). In our study, we did not perform RNA-seq of BRD4-KD cells, so we could not quantitatively assess the similarity of BRDT and BRD4 with regard to gene regulation. Such an experiment would be helpful for comprehensively uncovering the relation between BRDT and BRD4.

Another similarity between BRD4 and BRDT is the high Serine content in their CTDs. Interestingly, the Serine-rich CTD of BRD4 is intrinsically disordered and has been reported to participate in phase separation at super enhancers to promote gene expression (Sabari et al., 2018). A growing number of factors, such as RNA Pol II (Boehning et al., 2018), OCT4 and GCN4 (Boija et al., 2018), have been shown to promote phase separation. Because of the sequence similarity of the CTDs of BRD4 and BRDT and because the CTD of BRD4 is known to be intrinsically disordered, we tested whether BRDT also contains intrinsically disordered regions (IDRs). Expectedly, we found an IDR located within the CTD of BRDT (Fig. 24), hinting that BRDT could also help to from phase-separated condensates.

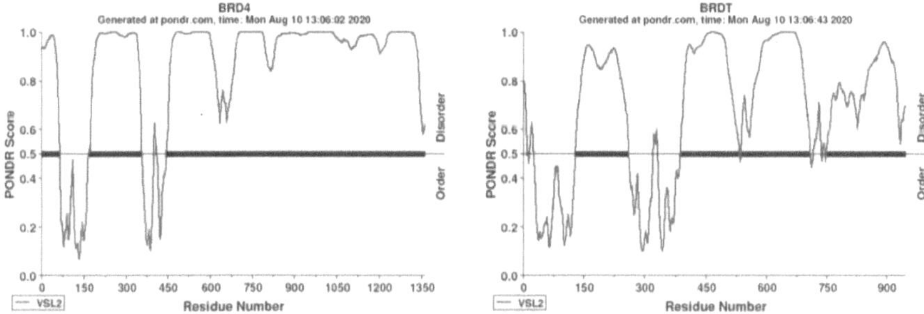

Fig. 24 IDR of BRD4 and BRDT identified by PONDR (Predicator of naturally disorder regions,

Besides the sequence similarity, we also found that BRD4 and BRDT co-localize with one another (Fig. 25 and Fig. 21C), especially at super enhancers, known hotspots for phase separated condensates. The sequence similarity and co-localization of BRD4 and BRDT prompted us to postulate that BRDT could also regulate gene expression through phase separation, most likely at super enhancers. We tested the effect of 1,6-hexanediol, a chemical which interrupts phase separation, on the expression of some genes driven by super enhancers. Interestingly, we found that a brief treatment with 1,6-hexanediol dramatically decreased the expression of MYC, suggesting that interrupting phase separation has a direct influence on transcription at certain genomic regions. However, these are just preliminary results and the role of BRDT, if there is any at all, in phase separation should be further studied.

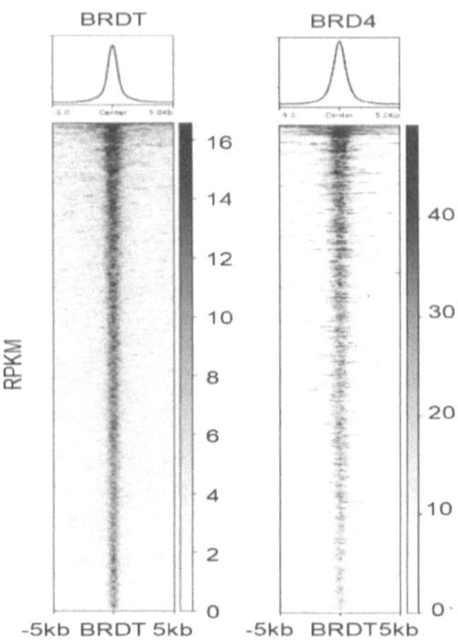

Fig. 25 The occupancy of BRDT and BRD4 on BRDT binding sites. The region is sorted by BRDT signal intensity. RPKM (reads per kilobase per million mapped reads).

Although there are a lot of similarities between BRD4 and BRDT, we should not ignore the difference between them. As we stated before, we did not perform RNA-seq following the knock-down of BRD4 in ESCC cell lines, so we cannot compare their target genes. However, the comparison between the binding sites of BRDT and BRD4 revealed some differences. Although both proteins co-localize in various genomic regions, BRDT and BRD4 also have some unique binding sites (34% for BRDT and 42% for BRD4, Fig. 26A). The difference between bromodomains is likely the cause of the differential binding of BRDT and BRD4. It is also worth noting that the regions, where BRD4 and BRDT co-localize have a higher signal intensity of both proteins compared with regions bound by just one of the BET proteins (Fig. 26B). BET proteins are typically recognized as positive transcription regulators, so the aforementioned result suggests that regions bound by both BRD4 and BRDT are generally more active compared with regions uniquely bound by either BRD4 or BRDT. As a confirmation of that, we found that 87% (277 out of 317) of the super enhancers called by BRDT were also identified by BRD4 (Fig. 21B). Our focus in this project was mostly put on the overlapped super enhancers while the region bound only by BRD4 or BRDT remains to be investigated.

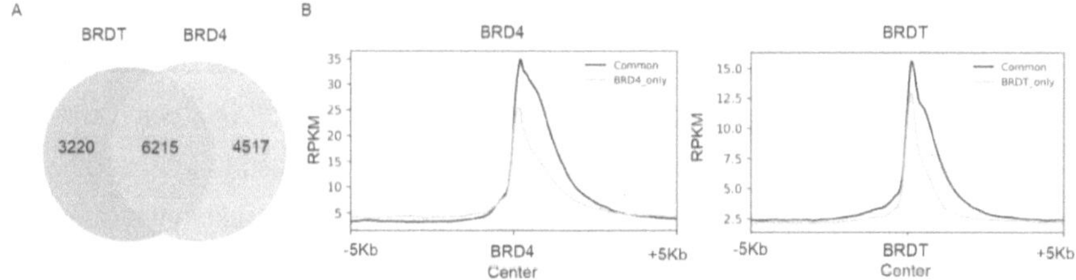

Fig. 26 Comparison of the occupancy of BRDT and BRD4. A: Venn diagram showing the overlap between BRDT binding sites and BRD4 binding sites; B: BRD4 (left) and BRDT (right) signal on regions bound by both BET proteins, BRD4 alone or BRDT alone.

Another interesting phenomenon that we observed was that the loss of BRDT disrupts the binding of BRD4 at some super enhancers. More specifically, we tested the binding of BRD4 upon depleting BRDT via siRNA-mediated knock-down and the binding of BRDT upon depleting BRD4. The binding of BRD4 at super enhancer sites, such as the *FAT2* super enhancer, significantly decreased upon the loss of BRDT. Neither BRDT nor BRD4 has any defined DNA-binding motif, such that they could be probably recruited to chromatin simultaneously. Since they are both transcriptional regulators, they should have reciprocal effects on one another. Unfortunately, that was not the case in our hands, as no decrease in BRDT binding at the *FAT2* super enhancer locus upon loss of BRD4 was observed. This seemed to propose a hierarchy of BRD4 and BRDT (at least at certain super enhancers) binding in which BRDT acts upstream of BRD4 and is likely to help recruit BRD4 to super enhancers. However, these are only preliminary results and more experiments are required to clarify the hierarchy. Taken together, BRDT and BRD4 share many similarities while retain their uniqueness.

3.4 ΔNp63: An active transcription factor without a transactivation domain

The transcription factor p63 was initially discovered as a p53 homolog for (Osada et al., 1998; Schmale and Bamberger, 1997; Trink et al., 1998) and it was recognized as an important transcription factor for epidermal development (Mills et al., 1999; Yang et al., 1999). The finding of more isoforms of p63 has led people to acknowledge its diversified function in development and disease progression. As previously mentioned, p63 mainly has two isoform categories arising from alternate TSSs: TAp63 and ΔNp63. TAp63 highly resembles its homolog p53 and it is also seen as a tumor suppressor because of its role in DNA damage response (Yang and McKeon, 2000). TAp63 is strongly expressed in oocytes and it protects the female germ line by promoting the elimination of oocytes that undergo DNA damage (Suh et al., 2006), being called the "guardian" of human reproduction (Amelio et al., 2012). Related to that, another p63 isoform, GTAp63, containing the transactivation domain was found in the male germ line. Similar to the function of TAp63 in oocytes, GTAp63 can induce apoptosis upon DNA damage in testes (Beyer et al., 2011). In our project, we showed a strong co-localization of ΔNp63 and BRDT, leading to a functional interplay between them. And the cooperation between these two proteins are important for some cellular processes such as cell migration. Given the testis-specific expression pattern of both GTAp63 and BRDT, it is possible that these two proteins work together to protect the genomic integrity in testes. Further experiments are required to test this hypothesis.

The transcriptional regulation of TAp63 or GTAp63 can largely be attributed to the TA domain, but if the TA domain is lost, would p63 lacking a TA domain (i.e. ΔNp63) become transcriptionally "silent"? It does not seem to be the case. For example, genetic depletion of p63 in mice and mutation of p63 in humans both lead to severe development defects which often occurs at sites dominated by the ΔNp63 isoform (Celli et al., 1999; Yang et al., 1999). This suggests that ΔNp63 is definitely functional and indispensable for normal development. Moreover, the expression of ΔNp63 is also altered in multiple cancers such as head and neck (Lo Muzio et al., 2005), breast (Tse et al., 2006) and lung cancer (Massion et al., 2003). A recent publication from our group also highlighted the role of ΔNp63 in forming an interconnected transcriptional network contributing the aggressiveness of a subgroup of PDAC (Hamdan and Johnsen, 2018). In squamous cell carcinoma, ΔNp63 has been shown to interact with SOX2 (Watanabe et al., 2014), or promote super enhancer-driven genes (*CCAT1* and *LINC01503*) (Jiang et al., 2018; Xie et al., 2018) to maintain the squamous lineage specification. In this project, we found that ΔNp63 is co-localized with BRDT and they positively regulate a common set of genes which are important for cell migration. These findings confirmed that ΔNp63 is active and contributes to squamous lineage maintenance in ESCC.

Interestingly, we noticed that although ΔNp63 has a lot of binding sites (37,730) along the genome, only a small portion of them are indeed active, i.e. marked by the active transcription mark, H3K27ac. For example, at the super enhancer site of *FAT2*, ΔNp63 is positioned exactly at the nucleosome-free region (NFR) and is surrounded by H3K27ac (Fig. 27A), indicating that this region is transcriptionally active. This is an example supporting our conclusion: ΔNp63 is an active transcription factor. However, there are also other inactive, but little or no H3K27ac (Fig. 27B), suggesting that ΔNp63 may also have a repressive role in ESCC.

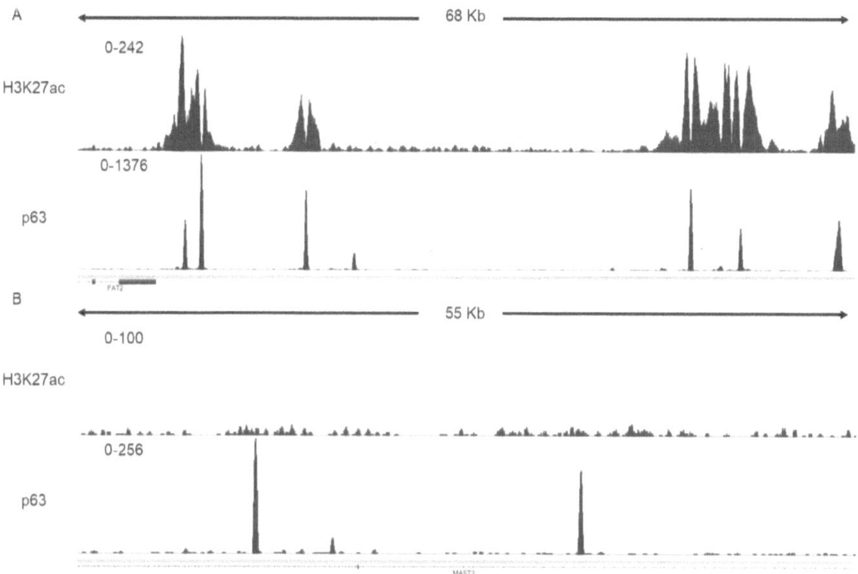

Fig. 27 Examples of active and inactive p63 sites. A: A region occupied by ΔNp63 and H3K27ac; B: A region occupied by ΔNp63 but devoid of H3K27ac.

Across the genome, only 32% of p63 binding sites overlap with H3K27ac, and even when extending p63 peaks by 2 Kb up- and downstream, the overlap between p63 and H3K27ac only increases by 8% (Fig. 28A). These results suggest that although ΔNp63 may bind to some genomic regions such as super enhancers to positively regulate oncogenic programs, it may still bind elsewhere to repress the gene expression. Indeed, the repressive role of ΔNp63 has been reported in various contexts (Mardaryev et al., 2016; De Rosa et al., 2009). To test if these sites are indeed repressed, we checked the signal of H3K27ac and H3K27me3 on active ΔNp63 sites (overlapped with H3K27ac) and inactive ΔNp63 sites (not overlapped with H3K27ac). The results showed that inactive ΔNp63 sites are marked by slightly higher level of H3K27me3 (Fig. 28B), indicating that these regions are possibly repressed.

However, this could also be a consequence of competition for the same substrate: H3K27. Because these inactive regions are devoid of H3K27ac, tri-methylation of H3K27 would be more likely to occur. However, the sigal intensity is really low for H3K27me3 and this may or may not have any biological function. Therefore, further experiments are required to characterize the inactive binding sites of p63 to better decipher the repressive role of ΔNp63 in ESCC.

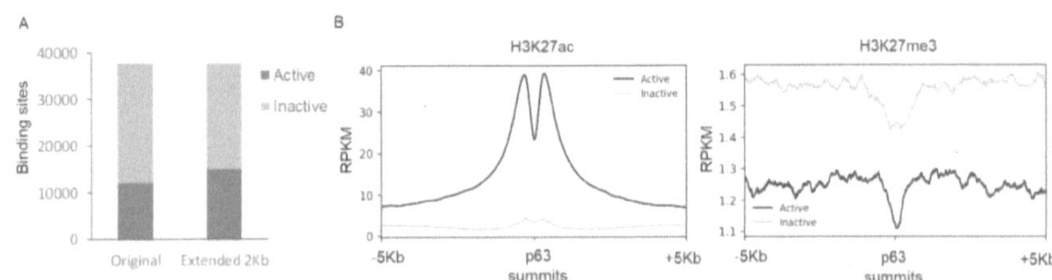

Fig. 28 Genome-wide analysis of p63 binding sites. A: Active and inactive binding sites of ΔNp63 in KYSE180; B: H3K27ac (left) and H3K27me3 (right) at active and inactive ΔNp63 summits.

3.5 Characterizing enhancers, super enhancers and their targets

Enhancers are regulatory elements that are marked by H3K27ac and H3K4me1 (Barski et al., 2007; Local et al., 2018; Pokholok et al., 2005). H3K4me3 is acknowledged as an active histone mark for transcription which locates in close proximity to promoters (Zhao et al., 2007). Taken these results together, it is widely accepted that regions marked by H3K27ac and H3K4me1 are active enhancers whereas regions marked by H3K27ac and H3K4me3 are active TSS̓s. However, admitting that this conclusion may apply to the majority of the regions, we found that it might not be accurate in some occasions. The association of H3K4me3 with enhancers has also been reported by several groups (Chen et al., 2015a; Pekowska et al., 2011). In this project, we also found some evidence which supports that H3K4me3 can also be associated with enhancers. For example, both the TSS and the associated super enhancer of *KRT14* are marked by both H3K4me1 and H3K4me3 marks (Fig. 29). These results stated that enhancers are not necessarily marked only by H3K4me1, but can also be marked by both H3K4me1 and H3K4me3.

Interestingly, H3K4me3 can sometimes also be found on super enhancers, being linked to super enhancer transcriptional activity yielding eRNAs (Cao et al., 2017; Li et al., 2019). The function of eRNA has been reported (Cinghu et al., 2017; Kaikkonen et al., 2013; Kim et al., 2010; Meng et al., 2014), but the detailed mechanism remains unclear. The exceptionally strong transcriptional activity of certain super enhancers can provide a unique opportunity for studying the mechanism underlying eRNA-mediated transcriptional regulation. In ESCC cells, we also found H3K4me3 signal at super enhancer sites, such as the super enhancer associated with *KRT14* (Fig. 29, in red rectangle), but whether eRNA is involved in BRDT- and ΔNp63-dependent transcriptional changes is yet to be answered.

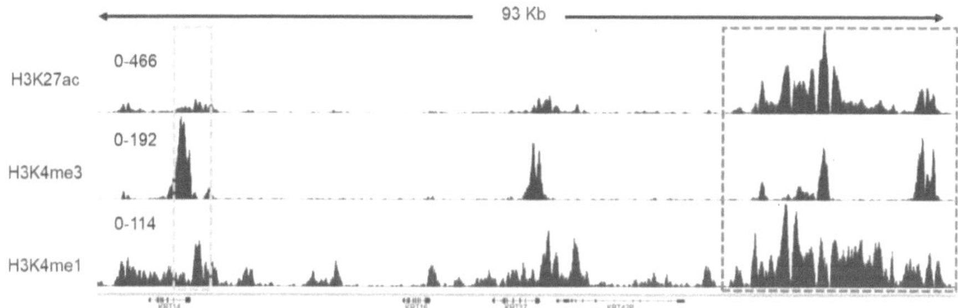

Fig. 29 An example of regions marked by H3K4me1 and H3K4me3. Yellow rectangle: TSS-proximal region of KRT14; Red rectangle: super enhancer associated with KRT14.

Another aspect to be considered when studying and characterizing super enhancers is the calling method of the latter. Super enhancers are clusters of active enhancers spanning a long stretch of genome, which mainly control genes associated with lineage specification and cell identity (Hnisz et al., 2013, 2014). In the context of cancer, super enhancers activate some oncogenes or oncogenic pathways to promote cancer progression (Hnisz et al., 2015; Lovén et al., 2013; Nakamura et al., 2017). Therefore, it is important to systematically identify super enhancers. The most widely-used method is ROSE (ranking of super enhancers) (Lovén et al., 2013; Whyte et al., 2013) which is also used in our study. However, the algorithm used by ROSE can introduce some bias by using an arbitrary cut-off. More specifically, ROSE merges H3K27ac peaks within 12.5 Kb. In other words, if two loci marked by H3K27ac are 13 Kb apart from one another, then they would not be considered for subsequent super enhancer-analysis, which could lead to a false negative result. More recently, CREAM (clustering of genomic regions analysis method) was developed and this tool took the variable distance between individual enhancers into consideration, which addressed the concern caused by using an arbitrary threshold. But it disqualifies all single enhancers which can span a big genomic region and act as a bona fide super enhancer, introducing potential biases (Tonekaboni et al., 2019). This highlights the need for a more comprehensive and unbiased tool for identifying super enhancers.

Given that we were mostly interested in BRDT-bound super enhancers, identifying super enhancer-associated genes became necessary. The widely used method for identifying genes associated with distal regulatory elements is based on directly picking the nearest genes up- and downstream from the region of interest. The online tool GREAT (genomic regions enrichment of annotations tool) can identify genes associated with enhancers including typical enhancers and super enhancers (McLean et al., 2010). It is a great tool but it can miss some important target genes that are not directly adjacent to the tested enhancers. Enhancers can form a loop to bring their targets into close proximity which means the actual target gene can be separated by several other genes in between. Therefore, methods based solely on linear distance can be misleading in certain cases. For example, if we choose GREAT, we would assign *KRT42P* (Keratin 42 Pseudogene) as the target of the *KRT14*-associated super enhancer. But *KRT42P* is not even expressed in our cell line, suggesting that it is probably not the actual target. In order to precisely map the gene-enhancer contact, we utilized a HiC-based method: HiChIP (Mumbach et al., 2016). Because enhancers are marked by H3K27ac, we used the antibody against H3K27ac to enrich for H3K27ac-associated chromatin contacts. Indeed, HiChIP for H3K27ac has helped us significantly to identify super enhancer-associated genes. An obvious example was that we were able to assign the super enhancer located at upstream of *KRT42P* to *KRT14* (Fig. 21C). In our study, we did not experimentally test the essentiality of BRDT-bound super enhancers in mediating transcriptional regulation. A nice validation of our chromatin interaction data would be to test the effects of inactivation or deletion of super enhancers on target gene expression using CRISPR/Cas9 (clustered regularly interspaced short palindromic repeats/Cas9)-based methods (Cong et al., 2013; Gilbert et al., 2013).

3.6 Clinical implications: BRDT-specific inhibitor/degrader and beyond

Our findings have established BRDT as an oncogenic protein with a role in promoting cell migration in ESCC. We further showed that BRDT acts at super enhancers to regulate genes that are important for phenotypic changes. This has rationalized the application of compounds specifically targeting super enhancers in cancers. In fact, the targeting of super enhancers has been tested in multiple cancer and gained some encouraging results *in vitro*. More specifically, CDK7 inhibition was the main strategy used to target super enhancers and has been proven to confer anti-tumor effects in osteosarcoma (Zhang et al., 2020b), neuroblastoma (Chipumuro et al., 2014) and nasopharyngeal carcinoma (Yuan et al., 2017). However, since our initial motivation was to identify a therapeutic target for potential applications in the scope of precision medicine, targeting super enhancers will probably affect other cells which are dependent on super enhancers as well, potentially leading to severe side effects. Instead, we suggest the targeting of BRDT as an alternative to targeting super enhancers, as we identify its tissue-specific expression and its role in ΔNp63-driven super enhancers.

The first BET inhibitors, such as JQ1 (Filippakopoulos et al., 2010), did not discriminate between the bromodomains of BRD2, BRD3, BRD4 and BRDT. Since then, significant advances have been made in this field over the last years. Now bromodomain-specific inhibition is possible and has shown different effects compared with pan-BET inhibitors. For example, ABBV-744, a compound specifically targeting the second bromodomain of BET proteins, showed decreased gastrointestinal toxicities when compare to pan-BET inhibitors (Faivre et al., 2020). Several groups are currently working on generating a BRDT-specific inhibitor for a completely different intention: male contraception. Therefore, specific targeting of BRDT may be feasible and could expectedly minimize side effects elicited by pan-BET inhibition.

BET proteins have multiple domains including bromodomains, extra-terminal domains and C-terminal domains, which diversify the function of BET proteins. For instance, in breast cancer while resistance to BET bromodomain inhibition was observed, the depletion of BRD4 could attenuate cell proliferation, suggesting that cells are likely to utilize BET proteins in a bromodomain-independent manner to survive (Shu et al.,

2016). In our study, we also found that some BRDT target genes, such as *KDM1B*, did not respond to BET inhibition, suggesting that BRDT has bromodomain-independent function. Therefore, pharmacologically degrading BET proteins represents a more attractive strategy. We tested a PROTAC (MZ1) which specifically degrades BET proteins. Indeed, it was able to rapidly degrade BET proteins (Chapter, Fig. 6E) and the degradation also led to altered gene expression resembling the knock-down of BRDT (Chapter, Fig. 6F). This is very encouraging because MZ1 already showed a BRDT specificity to some extent, suggesting the feasibility of developing a BRDT-specific PROTAC.

However, there is still a remaining question: would targeting a protein that has no effects on cell proliferation really bring clinical benefits? To maximize the value of BRDT-specific inhibitor, conjugating BRDT-specific inhibitor to other agents represents a reasonable strategy. Such theranostic methods have been explored in prostate cancer (Han et al., 2014) and breast cancer (Vultos et al., 2017) and have shown great potential for diagnosis and treatment. To exploit the clinical potential of BRDT, we can conjugate BRDT-specific inhibitor with an anti-tumor agent and the resulting hybrid compound would probably display strong anti-tumor effects in BRDT-expressing cells while spare the adjacent normal tissue without the expression of BRDT. And if the conjugating agent is radiolabeled, the resulting hybrid would also be helpful for monitoring tumor proliferation using non-invasive imaging. However, these hypotheses are based on the development of BRDT-specific inhibitor and need to be carefully tested in preclinical models.

Furthermore, the ectopic expression of CTAs can be immunogenic, thus representing a unique chance for immunotherapy. For example, MAGEA1 and NY-ESO1 (Chen et al., 1997) exhibited high immunogenicity, thus emerging as top candidates for immunotherapy. The clinical trial involving NY-ESO1 has yielded encouraging results with half of the enrolled patients showing tumor shrinkage (D'angelo et al., 2018). Moreover, many CTAs have been proven to promote cancer progression through different mechanisms as reviewed by Gibbs and Whitehurst (Gibbs and Whitehurst, 2018). Therefore, since BRDT has a cancer/testis-restricted expression pattern, its expression may evoke a T-cell mediated immune response. Unfortunately, there is no existing knowledge as to the immunogenicity of BRDT in cancer cells. Therefore, the role of BRDT in immune response should be further investigated to assess its potential for acting as an immunotherapeutic target. Overall, BRDT possesses a good clinical potential which should be further studied and tested in preclinical models.

3.7 Concluding remarks

To date, there are no effective target therapies for ESCC, a deadly malignancy with a 5-year survival rate of 15 to 20%. Using an unbiased screening, we were able to identify BRDT as a novel therapeutic target potentially with minimal side effects. We found that BRDT, the testis-specific BET protein, is indeed expressed in multiple cancers including ESCC. We, for the first time, uncovered that BRDT is dispensable for proliferation but can promote cell migration in the context of cancer. To mechanistically understand how BRDT functions to regulate cell migration, we conducted a knock down of BRDT followed by RNA-seq and found that many ECM-related pathways were enriched, which could explain the decrease in cell migration upon BRDT loss. By analyzing genes that are regulated by BRDT, we found that many BRDT targets are also ΔNp63 targets, suggesting a functional interplay between BRDT and ΔNp63. Subsequently, genomic occupancy profiling of BRDT revealed its binding preference towards promoters and enhancers. Strikingly, the consensus sequence of p63 binding motif was found in BRDT bound region, which supported that BRDT was functionally related to ΔNp63. Further genomic and transcriptomic analyses showed that BRDT and ΔNp63 co-localize and regulate a common subset of target genes. Knock-down of ΔNp63 could phenocopy BRDT loss, suggesting that ΔNp63 and BRDT cooperate to regulate genes which are important for cell migration. More interestingly, the overexpression of BRDT enhanced the expression of a subset of ΔNp63 targets and increased cell migratory potential. Furthermore, we found that BRDT co-localized with ΔNp63 at certain super enhancers to regulate gene expression. Importantly, pharmacological degradation of BRDT using a PROTAC resembled the siRNA-mediated knock-down of BRDT, suggesting a feasible way for targeting BRDT. Taken together, our work uncovered the tumorigenic role of BRDT in ESCC, suggesting it as a potential therapeutic target in the treatment of ESCC patients.

3.8 Supplemental figures

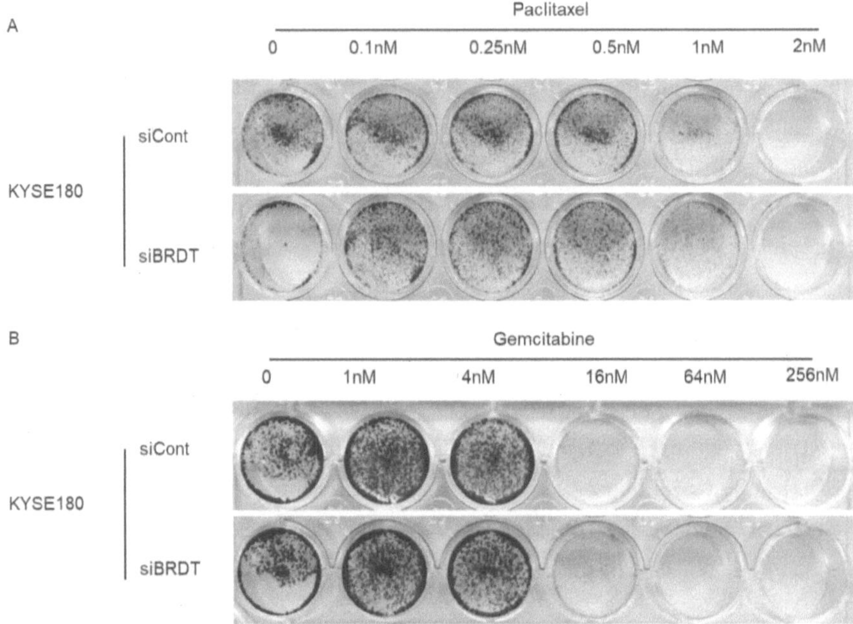

Fig. S4 Crystal violet staining showing cell proliferation upon Paclitaxel and Gemcitabine. Cells were treated with increasing concentrations of Paclitaxel and Gemcitabine for 48 hours after siRNA-mediated knock-down of BRDT.

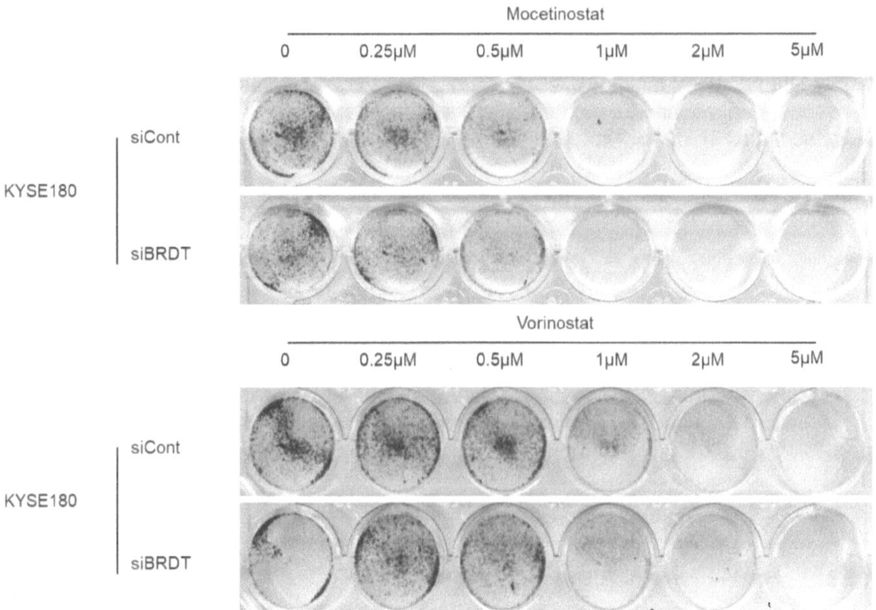

Fig. S5 Crystal violet staining showing cell proliferation upon HDAC inhibition. Cells were treated with increasing concentrations of Mocetinostat and Vorinostat for 48 hours after siRNA-mediated knock-down of BRDT.

References

Abnet, C.C., Wang, Z., Song, X., Hu, N., Zhou, F.-Y., Freedman, N.D., Li, X.-M., Yu, K., Shu, X.-O., Yuan, J.-M., et al. (2012). Genotypic variants at 2q33 and risk of esophageal squamous cell carcinoma in China: a meta-analysis of genome-wide association studies. Hum. Mol. Genet. *21*, 2132–2141.

Abnet, C.C., Arnold, M., and Wei, W.-Q. (2018). Epidemiology of Esophageal Squamous Cell Carcinoma. Gastroenterology *154*, 360–373.

Agger, K., Cloos, P.A.C., Christensen, J., Pasini, D., Rose, S., Rappsilber, J., Issaeva, I., Canaani, E., Salcini, A.E., and Helin, K. (2007). UTX and JMJD3 are histone H3K27 demethylases involved in HOX gene regulation and development. Nature *449*, 731–734.

Aird, F., Kandela, I., Mantis, C., Iorns, E., Denis, A., Williams, S.R., Perfito, N., and Errington, T.M. (2017). Replication study: BET bromodomain inhibition as a therapeutic strategy to target c-Myc. Elife *6*.

Alam, H., Tang, M., Maitituoheti, M., Dhar, S.S., Kumar, M., Han, C.Y., Ambati, C.R., Amin, S.B., Gu, B., Chen, T.Y., et al. (2020). KMT2D Deficiency Impairs Super-Enhancers to Confer a Glycolytic Vulnerability in Lung Cancer. Cancer Cell *37*, 599-617.e7.

Allfrey, V.G., Faulkner, R., and Mirsky, A.E. (1964). Acetylation and Methylation of Histones and Their Possible Role in the. Proc. Natl. Acad. Sci. United States *51*, 786–794.

Allum, W.H., Stenning, S.P., Bancewicz, J., Clark, P.I., and Langley, R.E. (2009). Long-term results of a randomized trial of surgery with or without preoperative chemotherapy in esophageal cancer. J. Clin. Oncol. *27*, 5062–5067.

Amelio, I., Grespi, F., Annicchiarico-Petruzzelli, M., and Melino, G. (2012). p63 the guardian of human reproduction. Cell Cycle *11*, 4545–4551.

Anders, S., Pyl, P.T., and Huber, W. (2015). HTSeq-A Python framework to work with high-throughput sequencing data. Bioinformatics *31*, 166–169.

Arias, J., Alberts, A.S., Brindle, P., Claret, F.X., Smeal, T., Karin, M., Feramisco, J., and Montminy, M. (1994). Activation of cAMP and mitogen responsive genes relies on a common nuclear factor. Nature *370*, 226–229.

Arnold, M., Soerjomataram, I., Ferlay, J., and Forman, D. (2015). Global incidence of oesophageal cancer by histological subtype in 2012. Gut *64*, 381–387.

Aronson, S.J., and Rehm, H.L. (2015). Building the foundation for genomics in precision medicine. Nature *526*, 336–342.

Arzate-Mejía, R.G., Josué Cerecedo-Castillo, A., Guerrero, G., Furlan-Magaril, M., and Recillas-Targa, F. (2020). In situ dissection of domain boundaries affect genome topology and gene transcription in Drosophila. Nat. Commun. *11*, 1–16.

Avilion, A.A., Nicolis, S.K., Pevny, L.H., Perez, L., Vivian, N., and Lovell-Badge, R. (2003). Multipotent cell lineages in early mouse development depend on SOX2 function. Genes Dev. *17*, 126–140.

Baedke, J. (2013). The epigenetic landscape in the course of time: Conrad Hal Waddington's methodological impact on the life sciences. Stud. Hist. Philos. Sci. Part C Stud. Hist. Philos. Biol. Biomed. Sci. *44*, 756–773.

Bai, L., Zhou, B., Yang, C.-Y., Ji, J., McEachern, D., Przybranowski, S., Jiang, H., Hu, J., Xu, F., Zhao, Y., et al. (2017). Targeted Degradation of BET Proteins in Triple-Negative Breast Cancer. Cancer Res. *77*, 2476–2487.

Bai, Y., Edamatsu, H., Maeda, S., Saito, H., Suzuki, N., Satoh, T., and Kataoka, T. (2004). Crucial role of phospholipase Cepsilon in chemical carcinogen-induced skin tumor development. Cancer Res. *64*, 8808–8810.

Bang, Y.-J., Van Cutsem, E., Feyereislova, A., Chung, H.C., Shen, L., Sawaki, A., Lordick, F., Ohtsu, A., Omuro, Y., Satoh, T., et al. (2010). Trastuzumab in combination with chemotherapy versus chemotherapy alone for treatment of HER2-positive advanced gastric or gastro-oesophageal junction cancer (ToGA): a phase 3, open-label, randomised controlled trial. Lancet (London, England) *376*, 687–697.

Bannister, A.J., Oehler, T., Wilhelm, D., Angel, P., and Kouzarides, T. (1995). Stimulation of c-Jun activity by CBP: c-Jun residues Ser63/73 are required for CBP induced stimulation in vivo and CBP binding in vitro. Oncogene *11*, 2509–2514.

Barretina, J., Caponigro, G., Stransky, N., Venkatesan, K., Margolin, A.A., Kim, S., Wilson, C.J., Lehár, J., Kryukov, G. V, Sonkin, D., et al. (2012). The Cancer Cell Line Encyclopedia enables predictive modelling of anticancer drug sensitivity. Nature *483*, 603–607.

Barski, A., Cuddapah, S., Cui, K., Roh, T.Y., Schones, D.E., Wang, Z., Wei, G., Chepelev, I., and Zhao, K. (2007). High-Resolution Profiling of Histone Methylations in the Human Genome. Cell *129*, 823–837.

Bass, A.J., Watanabe, H., Mermel, C.H., Yu, S., Perner, S., Verhaak, R.G., Kim, S.Y., Wardwell, L., Tamayo, P., Gat-Viks, I., et al. (2009). SOX2 is an amplified lineage-survival oncogene in lung and esophageal squamous cell carcinomas. Nat. Genet. *41*, 1238–1242.

Baylin, S.B., and Jones, P.A. (2016). Epigenetic determinants of cancer. Cold Spring Harb. Perspect. Biol. *8*.

Beagrie, R.A., Scialdone, A., Schueler, M., Kraemer, D.C.A., Chotalia, M., Xie, S.Q., Barbieri, M., De Santiago, I., Lavitas, L.M., Branco, M.R., et al. (2017). Complex multi-enhancer contacts captured by genome architecture mapping. Nature *543*, 519–524.

Bedenne, L., Michel, P., Bouché, O., Milan, C., Mariette, C., Conroy, T., Pezet, D., Roullet, B., Seitz, J.-F., Herr, J.-P., et al. (2007). Chemoradiation followed by surgery compared with chemoradiation alone in squamous cancer of the esophagus: FFCD 9102. J. Clin. Oncol. Off. J. Am. Soc. Clin. Oncol. *25*, 1160–1168.

Belinsky, S.A., Klinge, D.M., Stidley, C.A., Issa, J.P., Herman, J.G., March, T.H., and Baylin, S.B. (2003). Inhibition of DNA Methylation and Histone Deacetylation Prevents Murine Lung Cancer. Cancer Res. *63*, 7089–7093.

Belkhiri, A., and El-Rifai, W. (2015). Advances in targeted therapies and new promising targets in esophageal cancer. Oncotarget *6*, 1348–1358.

Belkina, A.C., and Denis, G. V. (2012). BET domain co-regulators in obesity, inflammation and cancer. Nat. Rev. Cancer *12*, 465–477.

Berndsen, C.E., Albaugh, B.N., Tan, S., and Denu, J.M. (2007). Catalytic mechanism of a MYST family histone acetyltransferase. Biochemistry *46*, 623–629.

Beyer, U., Moll-Rocek, J., Moll, U.M., and Dobbelstein, M. (2011). Endogenous retrovirus drives hitherto unknown proapoptotic p63 isoforms in the male germ line of humans and great apes. Proc. Natl. Acad. Sci. U. S. A. *108*, 3624–3629.

Bhattacharyya, S., Chandra, V., Vijayanand, P., and Ay, F. (2019). Identification of significant chromatin contacts from HiChIP data by FitHiChIP. Nat. Commun. *10*.

Bhutani, N., Brady, J.J., Damian, M., Sacco, A., Corbel, S.Y., and Blau, H.M. (2010). Reprogramming towards pluripotency requires AID-dependent DNA demethylation. Nature *463*, 1042–1047.

Bi, Y., Kong, P., Zhang, L., Cui, H., Xu, X., Chang, F., Yan, T., Li, J., Cheng, C., Song, B., et al. (2019). EP300 as an oncogene correlates with poor prognosis in esophageal squamous carcinoma. J. Cancer *10*, 5413–5426.

Bisgrove, D.A., Mahmoudi, T., Henklein, P., and Verdin, E. (2007). Conserved P-TEFb-interacting domain of BRD4 inhibits HIV transcription. Proc. Natl. Acad. Sci. U. S. A. *104*, 13690–13695.

Blaydon, D.C., Etheridge, S.L., Risk, J.M., Hennies, H.-C., Gay, L.J., Carroll, R., Plagnol, V., McRonald, F.E., Stevens, H.P., Spurr, N.K., et al. (2012). RHBDF2 mutations are associated with tylosis, a familial esophageal cancer syndrome. Am. J. Hum. Genet. *90*, 340–346.

Boehning, M., Dugast-Darzacq, C., Rankovic, M., Hansen, A.S., Yu, T., Marie-Nelly, H., McSwiggen, D.T., Kokic, G., Dailey, G.M., Cramer, P., et al. (2018). RNA polymerase II clustering through carboxy-terminal domain phase separation. Nat. Struct. Mol. Biol. *25*, 833–840.

Boija, A., Klein, I.A., Sabari, B.R., Dall'Agnese, A., Coffey, E.L., Zamudio, A. V., Li, C.H., Shrinivas, K., Manteiga, J.C., Hannett, N.M., et al. (2018). Transcription Factors Activate Genes through the Phase-Separation Capacity of Their Activation Domains. Cell *175*, 1842-1855.e16.

Bolden, J.E., Tasdemir, N., Dow, L.E., van Es, J.H., Wilkinson, J.E., Zhao, Z., Clevers, H., and Lowe, S.W. (2014). Inducible In Vivo Silencing of Brd4 Identifies Potential Toxicities of Sustained BET Protein Inhibition. Cell Rep. *8*, 1919–1929.

Boyes, J., Byfield, P., Nakatani, Y., and Ogryzko, V. (1998). Regulation of activity of the transcription factor GATA-1 by acetylation. Nature *396*, 594–598.

Bradner, J.E., Hnisz, D., and Young, R.A. (2017). Transcriptional Addiction in Cancer. Cell *168*, 629–643.

Brownell, J.E., Zhou, J., Ranalli, T., Kobayashi, R., Edmondson, D.G., Roth, S.Y., and Allis, C.D. (1996). Tetrahymena histone acetyltransferase A: A homolog to yeast Gcn5p linking histone acetylation to gene activation. Cell *84*, 843–851.

Bunney, T.D., Baxendale, R.W., and Katan, M. (2009). Regulatory links between PLC enzymes and Ras superfamily GTPases: signalling via PLCepsilon. Adv. Enzyme Regul. *49*, 54–58.

Bye, H., Prescott, N.J., Lewis, C.M., Matejcic, M., Moodley, L., Robertson, B., Rensburg, C. van, Parker, M.I., and Mathew, C.G. (2012). Distinct genetic association at the PLCE1 locus with oesophageal squamous cell carcinoma in the South African population. Carcinogenesis *33*, 2155–2161.

Cai, Y., Jin, J., Swanson, S.K., Cole, M.D., Choi, S.H., Florens, L., Washburn, M.P., Conaway, J.W., and Conaway, R.C. (2010). Subunit composition and substrate specificity of a MOF-containing histone acetyltransferase distinct from the Male-specific Lethal (MSL) complex. J. Biol. Chem. *285*, 4268–4272.

Cao, F., Fang, Y., Tan, H.K., Goh, Y., Choy, J.Y.H., Koh, B.T.H., Hao Tan, J., Bertin, N., Ramadass, A., Hunter, E., et al. (2017). Super-Enhancers and Broad H3K4me3 Domains Form Complex Gene Regulatory Circuits Involving Chromatin Interactions. Sci. Rep. *7*, 2186.

Celli, J., Duijf, P., Hamel, B.C.J., Bamshad, M., Kramer, B., Smits, A.P.T., Newbury-Ecob, R., Hennekam, R.C.M., Van Buggenhout, G., Van Haeringen, A., et al. (1999). Heterozygous germline mutations in the p53 homolog p63 are the cause of EEC syndrome. Cell *99*, 143–153.

Chen, E.Y., Tan, C.M., Kou, Y., Duan, Q., Wang, Z., Meirelles, G. V., Clark, N.R., and Ma'ayan, A. (2013). Enrichr: Interactive and collaborative HTML5 gene list enrichment analysis tool. BMC Bioinformatics *14*, 128.

Chen, H., Liu, H., and Qing, G. (2018). Targeting oncogenic Myc as a strategy for cancer treatment. Signal Transduct. Target. Ther. *3*, 5.

Chen, K., Chen, Z., Wu, D., Zhang, L., Lin, X., Su, J., Rodriguez, B., Xi, Y., Xia, Z., Chen, X., et al. (2015a). Broad H3K4me3 is associated with increased transcription elongation and enhancer activity at tumor-suppressor genes. Nat. Genet. *47*, 1149–1157.

Chen, T., Cheng, H., Chen, X., Yuan, Z., Yang, X., Zhuang, M., Lu, M., Jin, L., and Ye, W. (2015b). Family history of esophageal cancer increases the risk of esophageal squamous cell carcinoma. Sci. Rep. *5*, 16038.

Chen, Y.T., Scanlan, M.J., Sahin, U., Türeci, Ö., Gure, A.O., Tsang, S., Williamson, B., Stockert, E., Pfreundschuh, M., and Old, L.J. (1997). A testicular antigen aberrantly expressed in human cancers detected by autologous antibody screening.

Proc. Natl. Acad. Sci. U. S. A. *94*, 1914–1918.

Cheng, Z., Gong, Y., Ma, Y., Lu, K., Lu, X., Pierce, L.A., Thompson, R.C., Muller, S., Knapp, S., and Wang, J. (2013). Inhibition of BET bromodomain targets genetically diverse glioblastoma. Clin. Cancer Res. *19*, 1748–1759.

Chiang, C.M. (2014). Nonequivalent response to bromodomain-targeting BET inhibitors in oligodendrocyte cell fate decision. Chem. Biol. *21*, 804–806.

Chipumuro, E., Marco, E., Christensen, C.L., Kwiatkowski, N., Zhang, T., Hatheway, C.M., Abraham, B.J., Sharma, B., Yeung, C., Altabef, A., et al. (2014). Article CDK7 Inhibition Suppresses Super-Enhancer-Linked Oncogenic Transcription in MYCN-Driven Cancer. Cell *159*, 1126–1139.

Chrivia, J.C., Kwok, R.P., Lamb, N., Hagiwara, M., Montminy, M.R., and Goodman, R.H. (1993). Phosphorylated CREB binds specifically to the nuclear protein CBP. Nature *365*, 855–859.

Ciccone, D.N., Su, H., Hevi, S., Gay, F., Lei, H., Bajko, J., Xu, G., Li, E., and Chen, T. (2009). KDM1B is a histone H3K4 demethylase required to establish maternal genomic imprints. Nature *461*, 415–418.

Cinghu, S., Yang, P., Kosak, J.P., Conway, A.E., Kumar, D., Oldfield, A.J., Adelman, K., and Jothi, R. (2017). Intragenic Enhancers Attenuate Host Gene Expression. Mol. Cell *68*, 104-117.e6.

Clapier, C.R., Iwasa, J., Cairns, B.R., and Peterson, C.L. (2017). Mechanisms of action and regulation of ATP-dependent chromatin-remodelling complexes. Nat. Rev. Mol. Cell Biol. *18*, 407–422.

Cong, L., Ran, F.A., Cox, D., Lin, S., Barretto, R., Habib, N., Hsu, P.D., Wu, X., Jiang, W., Marraffini, L.A., et al. (2013). Multiplex genome engineering using CRISPR/Cas systems. Science (80-.). *339*, 819–823.

Consortium, E., Bernstein, B.E., Birney, E., Dunham, I., Green, E.D., Gunter, C., and Snyder, M. (2012). An integrated encyclopedia of DNA elements in the human genome. Nature *489*, 57–74.

Contrepois, K., Thuret, J.Y., Courbeyrette, R., Fenaille, F., and Mann, C. (2012). Deacetylation of H4-K16Ac and heterochromatin assembly in senescence. Epigenetics and Chromatin *5*, 15.

Creyghton, M.P., Cheng, A.W., Welstead, G.G., Kooistra, T., Carey, B.W., Steine, E.J., Hanna, J., Lodato, M.A., Frampton, G.M., Sharp, P.A., et al. (2010). Histone H3K27ac separates active from poised enhancers and predicts developmental state. Proc. Natl. Acad. Sci. U. S. A. *107*, 21931–21936.

Cui, R., Kamatani, Y., Takahashi, A., Usami, M., Hosono, N., Kawaguchi, T., Tsunoda, T., Kamatani, N., Kubo, M., Nakamura, Y., et al. (2009). Functional variants in ADH1B and ALDH2 coupled with alcohol and smoking synergistically enhance esophageal cancer risk. Gastroenterology *137*, 1768–1775.

Van Cutsem, E., Bang, Y.-J., Mansoor, W., Petty, R.D., Chao, Y., Cunningham, D., Ferry, D.R., Smith, N.R., Frewer, P., Ratnayake, J., et al. (2017). A randomized, open-label study of the efficacy and safety of AZD4547 monotherapy versus paclitaxel for the treatment of advanced gastric adenocarcinoma with FGFR2 polysomy or gene amplification. Ann. Oncol. Off. J. Eur. Soc. Med. Oncol. *28*, 1316–1324.

D'angelo, S.P., Melchiori, L., Merchant, M.S., Bernstein, D., Glod, J., Kaplan, R., Grupp, S., Tap, W.D., Chagin, K., Binder, G.K., et al. (2018). Antitumor activity associated with prolonged persistence of adoptively transferred NY-ESO-1c259T cells in synovial sarcoma. Cancer Discov. *8*, 944–957.

Dalgliesh, G.L., Furge, K., Greenman, C., Chen, L., Bignell, G., Butler, A., Davies, H., Edkins, S., Hardy, C., Latimer, C., et al. (2010). Systematic sequencing of renal carcinoma reveals inactivation of histone modifying genes. Nature *463*, 360–363.

Dang, C. V, O'Donnell, K.A., Zeller, K.I., Nguyen, T., Osthus, R.C., and Li, F. (2006). The c-Myc target gene network. Semin. Cancer Biol. *16*, 253–264.

Dawson, M.A., Kouzarides, T., and Huntly, B.J.P. (2012). Targeting epigenetic readers in cancer. N. Engl. J. Med. *367*, 647–657.

Dekker, J., Rippe, K., Dekker, M., and Kleckner, N. (2002). Capturing chromosome conformation. Science (80-.). *295*, 1306–1311.

Denis, G. V., McComb, M.E., Faller, D. V., Sinha, A., Romesser, P.B., and Costello, C.E. (2006). Identification of transcription complexes that contain the double bromodomain protein Brd2 and chromatin remodeling machines. J. Proteome Res. *5*, 502–511.

Denis, G. V, Vaziri, C., Guo, N., and Faller, D. V (2000). RING3 kinase transactivates promoters of cell cycle regulatory genes through E2F. Cell Growth Differ. Mol. Biol. J. Am. Assoc. Cancer Res. *11*, 417–424.

Devaiah, B.N., Lewis, B.A., Cherman, N., Hewitt, M.C., Albrecht, B.K., Robey, P.G., Ozato, K., Sims, R.J., and Singer, D.S. (2012). BRD4 is an atypical kinase that phosphorylates Serine2 of the RNA Polymerase II carboxy-terminal domain. Proc. Natl. Acad. Sci. U. S. A. *109*, 6927–6932.

Dhalluin, C., Carlson, J.E., Zeng, L., He, C., Aggarwal, A.K., and Zhou, M.M. (1999). Structure and ligand of a histone acetyltransferase bromodomain. Nature *399*, 491–496.

Dhar, S., Thota, A., and Rao, M.R.S. (2012). Insights into role of bromodomain, testis-specific (Brdt) in acetylated histone H4-dependent chromatin remodeling in mammalian spermiogenesis. J. Biol. Chem. *287*, 6387–6405.

Dobin, A., Davis, C.A., Schlesinger, F., Drenkow, J., Zaleski, C., Jha, S., Batut, P., Chaisson, M., and Gingeras, T.R. (2013). STAR: Ultrafast universal RNA-seq aligner. Bioinformatics *29*, 15–21.

Doi, T., Piha-Paul, S.A., Jalal, S.I., Mai-Dang, H., Saraf, S., Koshiji, M., Csiki, I., and

Bennouna, J. (2016). Updated results for the advanced esophageal carcinoma cohort of the phase 1b KEYNOTE-028 study of pembrolizumab. J. Clin. Oncol. *34*, 4046–4046.

Dostie, J., Richmond, T.A., Arnaout, R.A., Selzer, R.R., Lee, W.L., Honan, T.A., Rubio, E.D., Krumm, A., Lamb, J., Nusbaum, C., et al. (2006). Chromosome Conformation Capture Carbon Copy (5C): A massively parallel solution for mapping interactions between genomic elements. Genome Res. *16*, 1299–1309.

Doyle, J.M., Gao, J., Wang, J., Yang, M., and Potts, P.R. (2010). MAGE-RING protein complexes comprise a family of E3 ubiquitin ligases. Mol. Cell *39*, 963–974.

Dutton, S.J., Ferry, D.R., Blazeby, J.M., Abbas, H., Dahle-Smith, A., Mansoor, W., Thompson, J., Harrison, M., Chatterjee, A., Falk, S., et al. (2014). Gefitinib for oesophageal cancer progressing after chemotherapy (COG): a phase 3, multicentre, double-blind, placebo-controlled randomised trial. Lancet Oncol. *15*, 894–904.

Edgar, R., Domrachev, M., and Lash, A.E. (2002). Gene Expression Omnibus: NCBI gene expression and hybridization array data repository. Nucleic Acids Res. *30*, 207–210.

el-Deiry, W.S., Tokino, T., Velculescu, V.E., Levy, D.B., Parsons, R., Trent, J.M., Lin, D., Mercer, W.E., Kinzler, K.W., and Vogelstein, B. (1993). WAF1, a potential mediator of p53 tumor suppression. Cell *75*, 817–825.

Ellis, A., Field, J.K., Field, E.A., Friedmann, P.S., Fryer, A., Howard, P., Leigh, I.M., Risk, J., Shaw, J.M., and Whittaker, J. (1994). Tylosis associated with carcinoma of the oesophagus and oral leukoplakia in a large Liverpool family--a review of six generations. Eur. J. Cancer. B. Oral Oncol. *30B*, 102–112.

Ernst, J., and Kellis, M. (2012). ChromHMM: automating chromatin-state discovery and characterization. Nat. Methods *9*, 215–216.

Faivre, E.J., McDaniel, K.F., Albert, D.H., Mantena, S.R., Plotnik, J.P., Wilcox, D., Zhang, L., Bui, M.H., Sheppard, G.S., Wang, L., et al. (2020). Selective inhibition of the BD2 bromodomain of BET proteins in prostate cancer. Nature *578*, 306–310.

Filippakopoulos, P., and Knapp, S. (2012). The bromodomain interaction module. FEBS Lett. *586*, 2692–2704.

Filippakopoulos, P., Qi, J., Picaud, S., Shen, Y., Smith, W.B., Fedorov, O., Morse, E.M., Keates, T., Hickman, T.T., Felletar, I., et al. (2010). Selective inhibition of BET bromodomains. Nature *468*, 1067–1073.

Filippakopoulos, P., Picaud, S., Mangos, M., Keates, T., Lambert, J.P., Barsyte-Lovejoy, D., Felletar, I., Volkmer, R., Müller, S., Pawson, T., et al. (2012). Histone recognition and large-scale structural analysis of the human bromodomain family. Cell *149*, 214–231.

Finnin, M.S., Donigian, J.R., and Pavletich, N.P. (2001). Structure of the histone deacetylase SIRT2. Nat. Struct. Biol. *8*, 621–625.

Fitzmaurice, C., Dicker, D., Pain, A., Hamavid, H., Moradi-Lakeh, M., MacIntyre, M.F., Allen, C., Hansen, G., Woodbrook, R., Wolfe, C., et al. (2015). The Global Burden of Cancer 2013. JAMA Oncol. *1*, 505–527.

Freedman, N.D., Abnet, C.C., Leitzmann, M.F., Mouw, T., Subar, A.F., Hollenbeck, A.R., and Schatzkin, A. (2007a). A prospective study of tobacco, alcohol, and the risk of esophageal and gastric cancer subtypes. Am. J. Epidemiol. *165*, 1424–1433.

Freedman, N.D., Park, Y., Subar, A.F., Hollenbeck, A.R., Leitzmann, M.F., Schatzkin, A., and Abnet, C.C. (2007b). Fruit and vegetable intake and esophageal cancer in a large prospective cohort study. Int. J. Cancer *121*, 2753–2760.

French, C.A. (2010). NUT midline carcinoma. Cancer Genet. Cytogenet. *203*, 16–20.

French, C.A., Ramirez, C.L., Kolmakova, J., Hickman, T.T., Cameron, M.J., Thyne, M.E., Kutok, J.L., Toretsky, J.A., Tadavarthy, A.K., Kees, U.R., et al. (2008). BRD-NUT oncoproteins: A family of closely related nuclear proteins that block epithelial differentiation and maintain the growth of carcinoma cells. Oncogene *27*, 2237–2242.

Fuchs, C.S., Doi, T., Jang, R.W., Muro, K., Satoh, T., Machado, M., Sun, W., Jalal, S.I., Shah, M.A., Metges, J.P., et al. (2018). Safety and efficacy of pembrolizumab monotherapy in patients with previously treated advanced gastric and gastroesophageal junction cancer: Phase 2 clinical KEYNOTE-059 trial. JAMA Oncol. *4*, 180013.

Furlong, E.E.M., and Levine, M. (2018). Developmental enhancers and chromosome topology. Science (80-.). *361*, 1341–1345.

Gammon, M.D., Schoenberg, J.B., Ahsan, H., Risch, H.A., Vaughan, T.L., Chow, W.H., Rotterdam, H., West, A.B., Dubrow, R., Stanford, J.L., et al. (1997). Tobacco, alcohol, and socioeconomic status and adenocarcinomas of the esophagus and gastric cardia. J. Natl. Cancer Inst. *89*, 1277–1284.

Gantt, S.L., Joseph, C.G., and Fierke, C.A. (2010). Activation and inhibition of histone deacetylase 8 by monovalent cations. J. Biol. Chem. *285*, 6036–6043.

Gao, P., Yang, X., Suo, C., Yuan, Z., Cheng, H., Zhang, Y., Jin, L., Lu, M., Chen, X., and Ye, W. (2018). Socioeconomic status is inversely associated with esophageal squamous cell carcinoma risk: results from a population-based case-control study in China. Oncotarget *9*, 6911–6923.

Gao, Y.-B.B., Chen, Z.-L.L., Li, J.-G.G., Hu, X.-D. Da, Shi, X.-J.J., Sun, Z.-M.M., Zhang, F., Zhao, Z.-R.R., Li, Z.-T.T., Liu, Z.-Y.Y., et al. (2014). Genetic landscape of esophageal squamous cell carcinoma. Nat. Genet. *46*, 1097–1102.

Gao, Y., Hu, N., Han, X., Giffen, C., Ding, T., Goldstein, A., and Taylor, P. (2009). Family history of cancer and risk for esophageal and gastric cancer in Shanxi, China. BMC Cancer *9*, 269.

Garcia-Ramirez, M., Rocchini, C., and Ausio, J. (1995). Modulation of chromatin folding by histone acetylation. J. Biol. Chem. *270*, 17923–17928.

Garidou, A., Tzonou, A., Lipworth, L., Signorello, L.B., Kalapothaki, V., and Trichopoulos, D. (1996). Life-style factors and medical conditions in relation to esophageal cancer by histologic type in a low-risk population. Int. J. Cancer *68*, 295–299.

Gatti, V., Fierro, C., Annicchiarico-Petruzzelli, M., Melino, G., and Peschiaroli, A. (2019). ΔNp63 in squamous cell carcinoma: defining the oncogenic routes affecting epigenetic landscape and tumour microenvironment. Mol. Oncol. *13*, 981–1001.

Gaucher, J., Boussouar, F., Montellier, E., Curtet, S., Buchou, T., Bertrand, S., Hery, P., Jounier, S., Depaux, A., Vitte, A.L., et al. (2012). Bromodomain-dependent stage-specific male genome programming by Brdt. EMBO J. *31*, 3809–3820.

Gibbs, Z.A., and Whitehurst, A.W. (2018). Emerging Contributions of Cancer/Testis Antigens to Neoplastic Behaviors. Trends in Cancer *4*, 701–712.

Gilan, O., Rioja, I., Knezevic, K., Bell, M.J., Yeung, M.M., Harker, N.R., Lam, E.Y.N.N., Chung, C.-W.C., Bamborough, P., Petretich, M., et al. (2020). Selective targeting of BD1 and BD2 of the BET proteins in cancer and immunoinflammation. Science *368*, 387–394.

Gilbert, L.A., Larson, M.H., Morsut, L., Liu, Z., Brar, G.A., Torres, S.E., Stern-Ginossar, N., Brandman, O., Whitehead, E.H., Doudna, J.A., et al. (2013). CRISPR-mediated modular RNA-guided regulation of transcription in eukaryotes. Cell *154*, 442.

Gilkes, D.M., Semenza, G.L., and Wirtz, D. (2014). Hypoxia and the extracellular matrix: Drivers of tumour metastasis. Nat. Rev. Cancer *14*, 430–439.

Ginsburg, G.S., and Phillips, K.A. (2018). Precision Medicine: From Science To Value. Health Aff. (Millwood). *37*, 694–701.

Gong, F., Chiu, L.-Y., Cox, B., Aymard, F., Clouaire, T., Leung, J.W., Cammarata, M., Perez, M., Agarwal, P., Brodbelt, J.S., et al. (2015). Screen identifies bromodomain protein ZMYND8 in chromatin recognition of transcription-associated DNA damage that promotes homologous recombination. Genes Dev. *29*, 197–211.

Gorkin, D.U., Leung, D., and Ren, B. (2014). The 3D genome in transcriptional regulation and pluripotency. Cell Stem Cell *14*, 762–775.

Goutsouliak, K., Veeraraghavan, J., Sethunath, V., De Angelis, C., Osborne, C.K., Rimawi, M.F., and Schiff, R. (2020). Towards personalized treatment for early stage HER2-positive breast cancer. Nat. Rev. Clin. Oncol. *17*, 233–250.

Grasso, C.S., Wu, Y.M., Robinson, D.R., Cao, X., Dhanasekaran, S.M., Khan, A.P., Quist, M.J., Jing, X., Lonigro, R.J., Brenner, J.C., et al. (2012). The mutational landscape of lethal castration-resistant prostate cancer. Nature *487*, 239–243.

Greer, E.L., and Shi, Y. (2012). Histone methylation: A dynamic mark in health, disease and inheritance. Nat. Rev. Genet. *13*, 343–357.

Gressner, O., Schilling, T., Lorenz, K., Schulze Schleithoff, E., Koch, A., Schulze-

Bergkamen, H., Lena, A.M., Candi, E., Terrinoni, A., Catani, M.V., et al. (2005). TAp63alpha induces apoptosis by activating signaling via death receptors and mitochondria. EMBO J. *24*, 2458–2471.

Gu, W., and Roeder, R.G. (1997). Activation of p53 sequence-specific DNA binding by acetylation of the p53 C-terminal domain. Cell *90*, 595–606.

Hahn, S. (2018). Phase Separation, Protein Disorder, and Enhancer Function. Cell *175*, 1723–1725.

Hamdan, F.H., and Johnsen, S.A. (2018). DeltaNp63-dependent super enhancers define molecular identity in pancreatic cancer by an interconnected transcription factor network. Proc. Natl. Acad. Sci. U. S. A. *115*, E12343–E12352.

Hamilton, E., and Infante, J.R. (2016). Targeting CDK4/6 in patients with cancer. Cancer Treat. Rev. *45*, 129–138.

Han, G., Kortylewicz, Z.P., Enke, T., and Baranowska-Kortylewicz, J. (2014). Co-targeting androgen receptor and DNA for imaging and molecular radiotherapy of prostate cancer: in vitro studies. Prostate *74*, 1634–1646.

Harper, J.W., Adami, G.R., Wei, N., Keyomarsi, K., and Elledge, S.J. (1993). The p21 Cdk-interacting protein Cip1 is a potent inhibitor of G1 cyclin-dependent kinases. Cell *75*, 805–816.

Hazzouri, M., Pivot-Pajot, C., Faure, A.K., Usson, Y., Pelletier, R., Sèle, B., Khochbin, S., and Rousseaux, S. (2000). Regulated hyperacetylation of core histones during mouse spermatogenesis: Involvement of histone-deacetylases. Eur. J. Cell Biol. *79*, 950–960.

Heintzman, N.D., Stuart, R.K., Hon, G., Fu, Y., Ching, C.W., Hawkins, R.D., Barrera, L.O., Van Calcar, S., Qu, C., Ching, K.A., et al. (2007). Distinct and predictive chromatin signatures of transcriptional promoters and enhancers in the human genome. Nat. Genet. *39*, 311–318.

Heintzman, N.D., Hon, G.C., Hawkins, R.D., Kheradpour, P., Stark, A., Harp, L.F., Ye, Z., Lee, L.K., Stuart, R.K., Ching, C.W., et al. (2009). Histone modifications at human enhancers reflect global cell-type-specific gene expression. Nature *459*, 108–112.

Heinz, S., Benner, C., Spann, N., Bertolino, E., Lin, Y.C., Laslo, P., Cheng, J.X., Murre, C., Singh, H., and Glass, C.K. (2010). Simple Combinations of Lineage-Determining Transcription Factors Prime cis-Regulatory Elements Required for Macrophage and B Cell Identities. Mol. Cell *38*, 576–589.

Hennies, H.C., Hagedorn, M., and Reis, A. (1995). Palmoplantar keratoderma in association with carcinoma of the esophagus maps to chromosome 17q distal to the keratin gene cluster. Genomics *29*, 537–540.

Hnisz, D., Abraham, B.J., Lee, T.I., Lau, A., Saint-André, V., Sigova, A.A., Hoke, H.A., and Young, R.A. (2013). Super-enhancers in the control of cell identity and disease. Cell *155*, 934–947.

Hnisz, D., Abraham, B., Lee, T., Lau, A., Saint-Andre, V., Sigova, A., Hoke, H., and Young, R. (2014). Transcriptional super-enhancers connected to cell identity and disease. Cell *155*, 1–24.

Hnisz, D., Schuijers, J., Lin, C.Y., Weintraub, A.S., Abraham, B.J., Lee, T.I., Bradner, J.E., and Young, R.A. (2015). Convergence of Developmental and Oncogenic Signaling Pathways at Transcriptional Super-Enhancers. Mol. Cell *58*, 362–370.

Højfeldt, J.W., Agger, K., and Helin, K. (2013). Histone lysine demethylases as targets for anticancer therapy. Nat. Rev. Drug Discov. *12*, 917–930.

Holliday, R., and Pugh, J.E. (1975). DNA Modification Mechanisms and Gene Activity during Development.

Huang, B., Yang, X.-D., Zhou, M.-M., Ozato, K., and Chen, L.-F. (2009). Brd4 Coactivates Transcriptional Activation of NF-κB via Specific Binding to Acetylated RelA. Mol. Cell. Biol. *29*, 1375–1387.

Huang, H., Zhang, J., Shen, W., Wang, X., Wu, J., Wu, J., and Shi, Y. (2007). Solution structure of the second bromodomain of Brd2 and its specific interaction with acetylated histone tails. BMC Struct. Biol. *7*.

Hubbard, S.R., and Miller, W.T. (2007). Receptor tyrosine kinases: mechanisms of activation and signaling. Curr. Opin. Cell Biol. *19*, 117–123.

Hughes, J.R., Roberts, N., Mcgowan, S., Hay, D., Giannoulatou, E., Lynch, M., De Gobbi, M., Taylor, S., Gibbons, R., and Higgs, D.R. (2014). Analysis of hundreds of cis-regulatory landscapes at high resolution in a single, high-throughput experiment. Nat. Genet. *46*, 205–212.

Hynes, R.O. (2014). Stretching the boundaries of extracellular matrix research. Nat. Rev. Mol. Cell Biol. *15*, 761–763.

Ilson, D.H., Kelsen, D., Shah, M., Schwartz, G., Levine, D.A., Boyd, J., Capanu, M., Miron, B., and Klimstra, D. (2011). A phase 2 trial of erlotinib in patients with previously treated squamous cell and adenocarcinoma of the esophagus. Cancer *117*, 1409–1414.

Imai, S.I., Armstrong, C.M., Kaeberlein, M., and Guarente, L. (2000). Transcriptional silencing and longevity protein Sir2 is an NAD-dependent histone deacetylase. Nature *403*, 795–800.

Islami, F., Boffetta, P., Ren, J.-S., Pedoeim, L., Khatib, D., and Kamangar, F. (2009a). High-temperature beverages and foods and esophageal cancer risk--a systematic review. Int. J. Cancer *125*, 491–524.

Islami, F., Pourshams, A., Nasrollahzadeh, D., Kamangar, F., Fahimi, S., Shakeri, R., Abedi-Ardekani, B., Merat, S., Vahedi, H., Semnani, S., et al. (2009b). Tea drinking habits and oesophageal cancer in a high risk area in northern Iran: population based case-control study. BMJ *338*, b929.

Issa, J.P.J. (2007). DNA methylation as a therapeutic target in cancer. Clin. Cancer

Res. *13*, 1634–1637.

Jameson, J.L., and Longo, D.L. (2015). Precision medicine - Personalized, problematic, and promising. N. Engl. J. Med. *372*, 2229–2234.

Jankowska, A.M., Makishima, H., Tiu, R. V., Szpurka, H., Huang, Y., Traina, F., Visconte, V., Sugimoto, Y., Prince, C., O'Keefe, C., et al. (2011). Mutational spectrum analysis of chronic myelomonocytic leukemia includes genes associated with epigenetic regulation: UTX,,EZH2,and DNMT3A. Blood *118*, 3932–3941.

Jansson, C., Johansson, A.L. V, Nyrén, O., and Lagergren, J. (2005). Socioeconomic factors and risk of esophageal adenocarcinoma: a nationwide Swedish case-control study. Cancer Epidemiol. Biomarkers Prev. a Publ. Am. Assoc. Cancer Res. Cosponsored by Am. Soc. Prev. Oncol. *14*, 1754–1761.

Jiang, Y.-X., Zhang, D.-W., Chen, Y., Sun, H.-H., Xu, S.-C., and Gao, H.-J. (2015). The characteristics of oesophageal squamous cell carcinoma: an analysis of 1317 cases in southeastern China. Contemp. Oncol. (Poznan, Poland) *19*, 137–141.

Jiang, Y., Jiang, Y.Y., Xie, J.J., Mayakonda, A., Hazawa, M., Chen, L., Xiao, J.F., Li, C.Q., Huang, M.L., Ding, L.W., et al. (2018). Co-activation of super-enhancer-driven CCAT1 by TP63 and SOX2 promotes squamous cancer progression. Nat. Commun. *9*.

Jiang, Y.W., Veschambre, P., Erdjument-Bromage, H., Tempst, P., Conaway, J.W., Conaway, R.C., and Kornberg, R.D. (1998). Mammalian mediator of transcriptional regulation and its possible role as an end-point of signal transduction pathways. Proc. Natl. Acad. Sci. U. S. A. *95*, 8538–8543.

Johnson, C.A., White, D.A., Lavender, J.S., O'Neill, L.P., and Turner, B.M. (2002). Human class I histone deacetylase complexes show enhanced catalytic activity in the presence of ATP and co-immunoprecipitate with the ATP-dependent chaperone protein Hsp70. J. Biol. Chem. *277*, 9590–9597.

Kaikkonen, M.U., Spann, N.J., Heinz, S., Romanoski, C.E., Allison, K.A., Stender, J.D., Chun, H.B., Tough, D.F., Prinjha, R.K., Benner, C., et al. (2013). Remodeling of the enhancer landscape during macrophage activation is coupled to enhancer transcription. Mol. Cell *51*, 310–325.

Kanno, T., Kanno, Y., LeRoy, G., Campos, E., Sun, H.-W., Brooks, S.R., Vahedi, G., Heightman, T.D., Garcia, B.A., Reinberg, D., et al. (2014). BRD4 assists elongation of both coding and enhancer RNAs by interacting with acetylated histones. Nat. Struct. Mol. Biol. *21*, 1047–1057.

Kantidze, O.L., Gurova, K. V., Studitsky, V.M., and Razin, S. V. (2020). The 3D Genome as a Target for Anticancer Therapy. Trends Mol. Med. *26*, 141–149.

Kaur, J., Daoud, A., and Eblen, S.T. (2019). Targeting Chromatin Remodeling for Cancer Therapy. Curr. Mol. Pharmacol. *12*, 215–229.

Kayser, S., Krzykalla, J., Elliott, M.A., Norsworthy, K., Gonzales, P., Hills, R.K., Baer, M.R., Ráčil, Z., Mayer, J., Novak, J., et al. (2017). Characteristics and outcome of patients with therapy-related acute promyelocytic leukemia front-line treated with or without arsenic trioxide. Leukemia *31*, 2347–2354.

Kim, J., Bowlby, R., Mungall, A.J., Robertson, A.G., Odze, R.D., Cherniack, A.D., Shih, J., Pedamallu, C.S., Cibulskis, C., Dunford, A., et al. (2017). Integrated genomic characterization of oesophageal carcinoma. Nature *541*, 169–175.

Kim, T.K., Hemberg, M., Gray, J.M., Costa, A.M., Bear, D.M., Wu, J., Harmin, D.A., Laptewicz, M., Barbara-Haley, K., Kuersten, S., et al. (2010). Widespread transcription at neuronal activity-regulated enhancers. Nature *465*, 182–187.

Kleff, S., Andrulis, E.D., Anderson, C.W., and Sternglanz, R. (1995). Identification of a gene encoding a yeast histone H4 acetyltransferase. J. Biol. Chem. *270*, 24674–24677.

Koga, F., Kawakami, S., Fujii, Y., Saito, K., Ohtsuka, Y., Iwai, A., Ando, N., Takizawa, T., Kageyama, Y., and Kihara, K. (2003). Impaired p63 expression associates with poor prognosis and uroplakin III expression in invasive urothelial carcinoma of the bladder. Clin. Cancer Res. an Off. J. Am. Assoc. Cancer Res. *9*, 5501–5507.

Kornberg, R.D. (1974). Chromatin structure: A repeating unit of histones and DNA. Science (80-.). *184*, 868–871.

Kudo, T., Hamamoto, Y., Kato, K., Ura, T., Kojima, T., Tsushima, T., Hironaka, S., Hara, H., Satoh, T., Iwasa, S., et al. (2017). Nivolumab treatment for oesophageal squamous-cell carcinoma: an open-label, multicentre, phase 2 trial. Lancet Oncol. *18*, 631–639.

Kumar-Sinha, C., and Chinnaiyan, A.M. (2018). Precision oncology in the age of integrative genomics. Nat. Biotechnol. *36*, 46–60.

Lagergren, J., Smyth, E., Cunningham, D., and Lagergren, P. (2017). Oesophageal cancer. Lancet *390*, 2383–2396.

Laird, P.W., Jackson-Grusby, L., Fazeli, A., Dickinson, S.L., Edward Jung, W., Li, E., Weinberg, R.A., and Jaenisch, R. (1995). Suppression of intestinal neoplasia by DNA hypomethylation. Cell *81*, 197–205.

Lamonica, J.M., Deng, W., Kadauke, S., Campbell, A.E., Gamsjaeger, R., Wang, H., Cheng, Y., Billin, A.N., Hardison, R.C., Mackay, J.P., et al. (2011). Bromodomain protein Brd3 associates with acetylated GATA1 to promote its chromatin occupancy at erythroid target genes. Proc. Natl. Acad. Sci. U. S. A. *108*, E159–E168.

Lan, Q., Hsiung, C.A., Matsuo, K., Hong, Y.-C., Seow, A., Wang, Z., Hosgood, H.D. 3rd, Chen, K., Wang, J.-C., Chatterjee, N., et al. (2012). Genome-wide association analysis identifies new lung cancer susceptibility loci in never-smoking women in Asia. Nat. Genet. *44*, 1330–1335.

Langmead, B., Trapnell, C., Pop, M., and Salzberg, S.L. (2009). Ultrafast and memory-efficient alignment of short DNA sequences to the human genome. Genome Biol. *10*, R25.

LeRoy, G., Rickards, B., and Flint, S.J. (2008). The Double Bromodomain Proteins Brd2 and Brd3 Couple Histone Acetylation to Transcription. Mol. Cell *30*, 51–60.

Levi, F., Pasche, C., Lucchini, F., Bosetti, C., Franceschi, S., Monnier, P., and La Vecchia, C. (2000). Food groups and oesophageal cancer risk in Vaud, Switzerland. Eur. J. Cancer Prev. Off. J. Eur. Cancer Prev. Organ. *9*, 257–263.

Levine, A.J., and Oren, M. (2009). The first 30 years of p53: growing ever more complex. Nat. Rev. Cancer *9*, 749–758.

Li, H., Handsaker, B., Wysoker, A., Fennell, T., Ruan, J., Homer, N., Marth, G., Abecasis, G., and Durbin, R. (2009a). The Sequence Alignment/Map format and SAMtools. Bioinformatics *25*, 2078–2079.

Li, M., Edamatsu, H., Kitazawa, R., Kitazawa, S., and Kataoka, T. (2009b). Phospholipase Cepsilon promotes intestinal tumorigenesis of Apc(Min/+) mice through augmentation of inflammation and angiogenesis. Carcinogenesis *30*, 1424–1432.

Li, Q.-L., Wang, D.-Y., Ju, L.-G., Yao, J., Gao, C., Lei, P.-J., Li, L.-Y., Zhao, X.-L., and Wu, M. (2019). The hyper-activation of transcriptional enhancers in breast cancer. Clin. Epigenetics *11*, 48.

Li, S., Qian, J., Yang, Y., Zhao, W., Dai, J., Bei, J.-X., Foo, J.N., McLaren, P.J., Li, Z., Yang, J., et al. (2012). GWAS identifies novel susceptibility loci on 6p21.32 and 21q21.3 for hepatocellular carcinoma in chronic hepatitis B virus carriers. PLoS Genet. *8*, e1002791.

Li, S.H., Lu, H.I., Huang, W.T., Tien, W.Y., Lan, Y.C., Lin, W.C., Tsai, H.T., and Chen, C.H. (2018). The prognostic significance of histone demethylase UTX in esophageal squamous cell carcinoma. Int. J. Mol. Sci. *19*.

Li, W., Notani, D., Ma, Q., Tanasa, B., Nunez, E., Chen, A.Y., Merkurjev, D., Zhang, J., Ohgi, K., Song, X., et al. (2013). Functional roles of enhancer RNAs for oestrogen-dependent transcriptional activation. Nature *498*, 516–520.

Liang, H., Fan, J.-H., and Qiao, Y.-L. (2017). Epidemiology, etiology, and prevention of esophageal squamous cell carcinoma in China. Cancer Biol. Med. *14*, 33–41.

Lieberman-Aiden, E., Van Berkum, N.L., Williams, L., Imakaev, M., Ragoczy, T., Telling, A., Amit, I., Lajoie, B.R., Sabo, P.J., Dorschner, M.O., et al. (2009). Comprehensive mapping of long-range interactions reveals folding principles of the human genome. Science (80-.). *326*, 289–293.

Lin, D.-C., Hao, J.-J., Nagata, Y., Xu, L., Shang, L., Meng, X., Sato, Y., Okuno, Y., Varela, A.M., Ding, L.-W., et al. (2014). Genomic and molecular characterization of esophageal squamous cell carcinoma. Nat. Genet. *46*, 467–473.

Lin, D.C., Wang, M.R., and Koeffler, H.P. (2018). Genomic and Epigenomic Aberrations in Esophageal Squamous Cell Carcinoma and Implications for Patients. Gastroenterology *154*, 374–389.

Lin, Y., Totsuka, Y., He, Y., Kikuchi, S., Qiao, Y., Ueda, J., Wei, W., Inoue, M., and Tanaka, H. (2013). Epidemiology of esophageal cancer in Japan and China. J. Epidemiol. *23*, 233–242.

Liu, L., Scolnick, D.M., Trievel, R.C., Zhang, H.B., Marmorstein, R., Halazonetis, T.D., and Berger, S.L. (1999). p53 Sites Acetylated In Vitro by PCAF and p300 Are Acetylated In Vivo in Response to DNA Damage. Mol. Cell. Biol. *19*, 1202–1209.

Liu, W., Cheng, S., Asa, S.L., and Ezzat, S. (2008a). The melanoma-associated antigen A3 mediates fibronectin-controlled cancer progression and metastasis. Cancer Res. *68*, 8104–8112.

Liu, X., Wang, L., Zhao, K., Thompson, P.R., Hwang, Y., Marmorstein, R., and Cole, P.A. (2008b). The structural basis of protein acetylation by the p300/CBP transcriptional coactivator. Nature *451*, 846–850.

Liu, X., Zhang, M., Ying, S., Zhang, C., Lin, R., Zheng, J., Zhang, G., Tian, D., Guo, Y., Du, C., et al. (2017). Genetic Alterations in Esophageal Tissues From Squamous Dysplasia to Carcinoma. Gastroenterology *153*, 166–177.

Local, A., Huang, H., Albuquerque, C.P., Singh, N., Lee, A.Y., Wang, W., Wang, C., Hsia, J.E., Shiau, A.K., Ge, K., et al. (2018). Identification of H3K4me1-associated proteins at mammalian enhancers. Nat. Genet. *50*, 73–82.

Love, M.I., Huber, W., and Anders, S. (2014). Moderated estimation of fold change and dispersion for RNA-seq data with DESeq2. Genome Biol. *15*.

Lovén, J., Hoke, H.A., Lin, C.Y., Lau, A., Orlando, D.A., Vakoc, C.R., Bradner, J.E., Lee, T.I., and Young, R.A. (2013). Selective inhibition of tumor oncogenes by disruption of super-enhancers. Cell *153*, 320–334.

Lu, S.H., Camus, A.M., Tomatis, L., and Bartsch, H. (1981). Mutagenicity of extracts of pickled vegetables collected in Linhsien County, a high-incidence area for esophageal cancer in Northern China. J. Natl. Cancer Inst. *66*, 33–36.

Lv, S., Ji, L., Chen, B., Liu, S., Lei, C., Liu, X., Qi, X., Wang, Y., Lai-Han Leung, E., Wang, H., et al. (2018). Histone methyltransferase KMT2D sustains prostate carcinogenesis and metastasis via epigenetically activating LIFR and KLF4. Oncogene *37*, 1354–1368.

Maine, E.A., Westcott, J.M., Prechtl, A.M., Dang, T.T., Whitehurst, A.W., and Pearson, G.W. (2016). The cancer-testis antigens SPANX-A/C/D and CTAG2 promote breast cancer invasion. Oncotarget *7*, 14708–14726.

Mann, B.S., Johnson, J.R., Cohen, M.H., Justice, R., and Pazdur, R. (2007). FDA Approval Summary: Vorinostat for Treatment of Advanced Primary Cutaneous T-Cell Lymphoma. Oncologist *12*, 1247–1252.

Mantovani, F., Collavin, L., and Del Sal, G. (2019). Mutant p53 as a guardian of the cancer cell. Cell Death Differ. *26*, 199–212.

Mardaryev, A.N., Liu, B., Rapisarda, V., Poterlowicz, K., Malashchuk, I., Rudolf, J.,

Sharov, A.A., Jahoda, C.A., Fessing, M.Y., Benitah, S.A., et al. (2016). Cbx4 maintains the epithelial lineage identity and cell proliferation in the developing stratified epithelium. J. Cell Biol. *212*, 77–89.

Margueron, R., Justin, N., Ohno, K., Sharpe, M.L., Son, J., Drury, W.J., Voigt, P., Martin, S.R., Taylor, W.R., De Marco, V., et al. (2009). Role of the polycomb protein EED in the propagation of repressive histone marks. Nature *461*, 762–767.

Marmorstein, R., and Zhou, M.M. (2014). Writers and readers of histone acetylation: Structure, mechanism, and inhibition. Cold Spring Harb. Perspect. Biol. *6*, a018762.

Massion, P.P., Taflan, P.M., Jamshedur Rahman, S.M., Yildiz, P., Shyr, Y., Edgerton, M.E., Westfall, M.D., Roberts, J.R., Pietenpol, J.A., Carbone, D.P., et al. (2003). Significance of p63 amplification and overexpression in lung cancer development and prognosis. Cancer Res. *63*, 7113–7121.

Matsui, S., Utani, A., Takahashi, K., Mukoyama, Y., Miyachi, Y., and Matsuyoshi, N. (2008). Knockdown of Fat2 by siRNA inhibits the migration of human squamous carcinoma cells. J. Dermatol. Sci. *51*, 207–210.

Matzuk, M.M., McKeown, M.R., Filippakopoulos, P., Li, Q., Ma, L., Agno, J.E., Lemieux, M.E., Picaud, S., Yu, R.N., Qi, J., et al. (2012). Small-molecule inhibition of BRDT for male contraception. Cell *150*, 673–684.

Mauro, M.J., O'Dwyer, M.E., and Druker, B.J. (2001). STI571, a tyrosine kinase inhibitor for the treatment of chronic myelogenous leukemia: Validating the promise of molecularly targeted therapy. Cancer Chemother. Pharmacol. *48*.

McLean, C.Y., Bristor, D., Hiller, M., Clarke, S.L., Schaar, B.T., Lowe, C.B., Wenger, A.M., and Bejerano, G. (2010). GREAT improves functional interpretation of cis-regulatory regions. Nat. Biotechnol. *28*, 495–501.

Meistrich, M.L., Trostle-Weige, P.K., Lin, R., Allis, C.D., and Bhatnagar, Y.M. (1992). Highly acetylated H4 is associated with histone displacement in rat spermatids. Mol. Reprod. Dev. *31*, 170–181.

Melino, G. (2011). P63 is a suppressor of tumorigenesis and metastasis interacting with mutant p53. Cell Death Differ. *18*, 1487–1499.

Meng, F.L., Du, Z., Federation, A., Hu, J., Wang, Q., Kieffer-Kwon, K.R., Meyers, R.M., Amor, C., Wasserman, C.R., Neuberg, D., et al. (2014). Convergent transcription at intragenic super-enhancers targets AID-initiated genomic instability. Cell *159*, 1538–1548.

Middleton, D.R., Menya, D., Kigen, N., Oduor, M., Maina, S.K., Some, F., Chumba, D., Ayuo, P., Osano, O., Schüz, J., et al. (2019). Hot beverages and oesophageal cancer risk in western Kenya: Findings from the ESCCAPE case–control study. Int. J. Cancer *144*, 2669–2676.

Miller, T.C.R., Simon, B., Rybin, V., Grötsch, H., Curtet, S., Khochbin, S., Carlomagno, T., and Müller, C.W. (2016). A bromodomain-DNA interaction facilitates acetylation-dependent bivalent nucleosome recognition by the BET protein BRDT.

Nat. Commun. *7*, 1–13.

Mills, A.A., Zheng, B., Wang, X.J., Vogel, H., Roop, D.R., and Bradley, A. (1999). p63 is a p53 homologue required for limb and epidermal morphogenesis. Nature *398*, 708–713.

Miyoshi, I., Aster, J.C., Kubonishi, I., Kroll, T.G., Dal Cin, P., Vargas, S.O., Perez-Atayde, A.R., and Fletcher, J.A. (2001). BRD4 bromodomain gene rearrangement in aggressive carcinoma with translocation t(15;19). Am. J. Pathol. *159*, 1987–1992.

Mizumoto, A., Ohashi, S., Hirohashi, K., Amanuma, Y., Matsuda, T., and Muto, M. (2017). Molecular Mechanisms of Acetaldehyde-Mediated Carcinogenesis in Squamous Epithelium. Int. J. Mol. Sci. *18*.

Monte, M., Simonatto, M., Peche, L.Y., Bublik, D.R., Gobessi, S., Pierotti, M.A., Rodolfo, M., and Schneider, C. (2006). MAGE-A tumor antigens target p53 transactivation function through histone deacetylase recruitment and confer resistance to chemotherapeutic agents. Proc. Natl. Acad. Sci. U. S. A. *103*, 11160–11165.

Montgomery, R.L., Davis, C.A., Potthoff, M.J., Haberland, M., Fielitz, J., Qi, X., Hill, J.A., Richardson, J.A., and Olson, E.N. (2007). Histone deacetylases 1 and 2 redundantly regulate cardiac morphogenesis, growth, and contractility. Genes Dev. *21*, 1790–1802.

Moon, K.J., Mochizuki, K., Zhou, M., Jeong, H.-S.S., Brady, J.N., Ozato, K., Jang, M.K., Mochizuki, K., Zhou, M., Jeong, H.-S.S., et al. (2005). The bromodomain protein Brd4 is a positive regulatory component of P-TEFb and stimulates RNA polymerase II-dependent transcription. Mol. Cell *19*, 523–534.

Morel, D., Jeffery, D., Aspeslagh, S., Almouzni, G., and Postel-Vinay, S. (2020). Combining epigenetic drugs with other therapies for solid tumours — past lessons and future promise. Nat. Rev. Clin. Oncol. *17*, 91–107.

Morinière, J., Rousseaux, S., Steuerwald, U., Soler-López, M., Curtet, S., Vitte, A.L., Govin, J., Gaucher, J., Sadoul, K., Hart, D.J., et al. (2009). Cooperative binding of two acetylation marks on a histone tail by a single bromodomain. Nature *461*, 664–668.

Moses, M.A., George, A.L., Sakakibara, N., Mahmood, K., Ponnamperuma, R.M., King, K.E., and Weinberg, W.C. (2019). Molecular mechanisms of p63-mediated squamous cancer pathogenesis. Int. J. Mol. Sci. *20*.

Mousavi, K., Zare, H., Dell'Orso, S., Grontved, L., Gutierrez-Cruz, G., Derfoul, A., Hager, G.L., and Sartorelli, V. (2013). ERNAs Promote Transcription by Establishing Chromatin Accessibility at Defined Genomic Loci. Mol. Cell *51*, 606–617.

Mujtaba, S., Zeng, L., and Zhou, M.M. (2007). Structure and acetyl-lysine recognition of the bromodomain. Oncogene *26*, 5521–5527.

Mumbach, M.R., Rubin, A.J., Flynn, R.A., Dai, C., Khavari, P.A., Greenleaf, W.J., and Chang, H.Y. (2016). HiChIP: Efficient and sensitive analysis of protein-directed genome architecture. Nat. Methods *13*, 919–922.

Munishi, M.O., Hanisch, R., Mapunda, O., Ndyetabura, T., Ndaro, A., Schüz, J., Kibiki, G., and McCormack, V. (2015). Africa's oesophageal cancer corridor: Do hot beverages contribute? Cancer Causes Control *26*, 1477–1486.

Munshi, N., Agalioti, T., Lomvardas, S., Merika, M., Chen, G., and Thanos, D. (2001). Coordination of a transcriptional switch by HMGI(Y) acetylation. Science (80-.). *293*, 1133–1136.

Murray-Zmijewski, F., Lane, D.P., and Bourdon, J.C. (2006). p53/p63/p73 isoforms: An orchestra of isoforms to harmonise cell differentiation and response to stress. Cell Death Differ. *13*, 962–972.

Lo Muzio, L., Santarelli, A., Caltabiano, R., Rubini, C., Pieramici, T., Trevisiol, L., Carinci, F., Leonardi, R., De Lillo, A., Lanzafame, S., et al. (2005). p63 overexpression associates with poor prognosis in head and neck squamous cell carcinoma. Hum. Pathol. *36*, 187–194.

Nagy, Z., Riss, A., Fujiyama, S., Krebs, A., Orpinell, M., Jansen, P., Cohen, A., Stunnenberg, H.G., Kato, S., and Tora, L. (2010). The metazoan ATAC and SAGA coactivator HAT complexes regulate different sets of inducible target genes. Cell. Mol. Life Sci. *67*, 611–628.

Nair, S.S., and Kumar, R. (2012). Chromatin remodeling in Cancer: A Gateway to regulate gene Transcription. Mol. Oncol. *6*, 611–619.

Najafova, Z., Tirado-Magallanes, R., Subramaniam, M., Hossan, T., Schmidt, G., Nagarajan, S., Baumgart, S.J., Mishra, V.K., Bedi, U., Hesse, E., et al. (2017). BRD4 localization to lineage-specific enhancers is associated with a distinct transcription factor repertoire. Nucleic Acids Res. *45*, 127–141.

Nakamura, Y., Hattori, N., Iida, N., Yamashita, S., Mori, A., Kimura, K., Yoshino, T., and Ushijima, T. (2017). Targeting of super-enhancers and mutant BRAF can suppress growth of BRAF-mutant colon cancer cells via repression of MAPK signaling pathway. Cancer Lett. *402*, 100–109.

Nickerson, M.L., Dancik, G.M., Im, K.M., Edwards, M.G., Turan, S., Brown, J., Ruiz-Rodriguez, C., Owens, C., Costello, J.C., Guo, G., et al. (2014). Concurrent alterations in TERT, KDM6A, and the BRCA pathway in bladder cancer. Clin. Cancer Res. *20*, 4935–4948.

Njei, B., McCarty, T.R., and Birk, J.W. (2016). Trends in esophageal cancer survival in United States adults from 1973 to 2009: A SEER database analysis. J. Gastroenterol. Hepatol. *31*, 1141–1146.

Ogryzko, V. V., Schiltz, R.L., Russanova, V., Howard, B.H., and Nakatani, Y. (1996). The transcriptional coactivators p300 and CBP are histone acetyltransferases. Cell *87*, 953–959.

Ohashi, S., Miyamoto, S., Kikuchi, O., Goto, T., Amanuma, Y., and Muto, M. (2015). Recent Advances From Basic and Clinical Studies of Esophageal Squamous Cell

Carcinoma. Gastroenterology *149*, 1700–1715.

Ohtsu, A., Shah, M.A., Van Cutsem, E., Rha, S.Y., Sawaki, A., Park, S.R., Lim, H.Y., Yamada, Y., Wu, J., Langer, B., et al. (2011). Bevacizumab in combination with chemotherapy as first-line therapy in advanced gastric cancer: a randomized, double-blind, placebo-controlled phase III study. J. Clin. Oncol. Off. J. Am. Soc. Clin. Oncol. *29*, 3968–3976.

Ohtsu, A., Ajani, J.A., Bai, Y.-X., Bang, Y.-J., Chung, H.-C., Pan, H.-M., Sahmoud, T., Shen, L., Yeh, K.-H., Chin, K., et al. (2013). Everolimus for previously treated advanced gastric cancer: results of the randomized, double-blind, phase III GRANITE-1 study. J. Clin. Oncol. Off. J. Am. Soc. Clin. Oncol. *31*, 3935–3943.

Okano, M., Xie, S., and Li, E. (1998). Cloning and characterization of a family of novel mammalian DNA (cytosine-5) methyltransferases. Nat. Genet. *19*, 219–220.

Okano, M., Bell, D.W., Haber, D.A., and Li, E. (1999). DNA methyltransferases Dnmt3a and Dnmt3b are essential for de novo methylation and mammalian development. Cell *99*, 247–257.

Okines, A., Cunningham, D., and Chau, I. (2011). Targeting the human EGFR family in esophagogastric cancer. Nat. Rev. Clin. Oncol. *8*, 492–503.

Osada, M., Ohba, M., Kawahara, C., Ishioka, C., Kanamaru, R., Katoh, I., Ikawa, Y., Nimura, Y., Nakagawara, A., Obinata, M., et al. (1998). Cloning and functional analysis of human p51, which structurally and functionally resembles p53. Nat. Med. *4*, 839–843.

Patel, A., Dharmarajan, V., Vought, V.E., and Cosgrove, M.S. (2009). On the mechanism of multiple lysine methylation by the human mixed lineage leukemia protein-1 (MLL1) core complex. J. Biol. Chem. *284*, 24242–24256.

Pekowska, A., Benoukraf, T., Zacarias-Cabeza, J., Belhocine, M., Koch, F., Holota, H., Imbert, J., Andrau, J.-C., Ferrier, P., and Spicuglia, S. (2011). H3K4 tri-methylation provides an epigenetic signature of active enhancers. EMBO J. *30*, 4198–4210.

Peng, J., Dong, W., Chen, L., Zou, T., Qi, Y., and Liu, Y. (2007). Brd2 is a TBP-associated protein and recruits TBP into E2F-1 transcriptional complex in response to serum stimulation. Mol. Cell. Biochem. *294*, 45–54.

Picaud, S., Wells, C., Felletar, I., Brotherton, D., Martin, S., Savitsky, P., Diez-Dacal, B., Philpott, M., Bountra, C., Lingard, H., et al. (2013). RVX-208, an inhibitor of BET transcriptional regulators with selectivity for the second bromodomain. Proc. Natl. Acad. Sci. U. S. A. *110*, 19754–19759.

Piha-Paul, S.A., Hann, C.L., French, C.A., Cousin, S., Braña, I., Cassier, P.A., Moreno, V., de Bono, J.S., Harward, S.D., Ferron-Brady, G., et al. (2020). Phase 1 Study of Molibresib (GSK525762), a Bromodomain and Extra-Terminal Domain Protein Inhibitor, in NUT Carcinoma and Other Solid Tumors. JNCI Cancer Spectr. *4*.

Pirrotta, V. (1998). Polycombing the genome: PcG, trxG and chromatin silencing.

Cell *93*, 333–336.

Pivot-Pajot, C., Caron, C., Govin, J., Vion, A., Rousseaux, S., and Khochbin, S. (2003). Acetylation-Dependent Chromatin Reorganization by BRDT, a Testis-Specific Bromodomain-Containing Protein Downloaded from. Mol. Cell. Biol. *23*, 5354–5365.

Pokholok, D.K., Harbison, C.T., Levine, S., Cole, M., Hannett, N.M., Tong, I.L., Bell, G.W., Walker, K., Rolfe, P.A., Herbolsheimer, E., et al. (2005). Genome-wide map of nucleosome acetylation and methylation in yeast. Cell *122*, 517–527.

Prabhu, A., Obi, K.O., and Rubenstein, J.H. (2014). The synergistic effects of alcohol and tobacco consumption on the risk of esophageal squamous cell carcinoma: a meta-analysis. Am. J. Gastroenterol. *109*, 822–827.

Prasad, V., Fojo, T., and Brada, M. (2016). Precision oncology: Origins, optimism, and potential. Lancet Oncol. *17*, e81–e86.

Rahman, S., Sowa, M.E., Ottinger, M., Smith, J.A., Shi, Y., Harper, J.W., and Howley, P.M. (2011). The Brd4 Extraterminal Domain Confers Transcription Activation Independent of pTEFb by Recruiting Multiple Proteins, Including NSD3. Mol. Cell. Biol. *31*, 2641–2652.

Raina, K., Lu, J., Qian, Y., Altieri, M., Gordon, D., Rossi, A.M.K., Wang, J., Chen, X., Dong, H., Siu, K., et al. (2016). PROTAC-induced BET protein degradation as a therapy for castration-resistant prostate cancer. Proc. Natl. Acad. Sci. U. S. A. *113*, 7124–7129.

Ramírez, F., Dündar, F., Diehl, S., Grüning, B.A., and Manke, T. (2014). DeepTools: A flexible platform for exploring deep-sequencing data. Nucleic Acids Res. *42*.

Rao, R.C., and Dou, Y. (2015). Hijacked in cancer: The KMT2 (MLL) family of methyltransferases. Nat. Rev. Cancer *15*, 334–346.

Rathke, C., Baarends, W.M., Awe, S., and Renkawitz-Pohl, R. (2014). Chromatin dynamics during spermiogenesis. Biochim. Biophys. Acta - Gene Regul. Mech. *1839*, 155–168.

Renaud, S., Loukinov, D., Alberti, L., Vostrov, A., Kwon, Y.W., Bosman, F.T., Lobanenkov, V., and Benhattar, J. (2011). BORIS/CTCFL-mediated transcriptional regulation of the hTERT telomerase gene in testicular and ovarian tumor cells. Nucleic Acids Res. *39*, 862–873.

Riboli, E., and Norat, T. (2003). Epidemiologic evidence of the protective effect of fruit and vegetables on cancer risk. Am. J. Clin. Nutr. *78*, 559S-569S.

Richardson, P.G., Laubach, J.P., Lonial, S., Moreau, P., Yoon, S.S., Hungria, V.T., Dimopoulos, M.A., Beksac, M., Alsina, M., and San-Miguel, J.F. (2015). Panobinostat: A novel pan-deacetylase inhibitor for the treatment of relapsed or relapsed and refractory multiple myeloma. Expert Rev. Anticancer Ther. *15*, 737–748.

Riggs, A.D. (1975). X inactivation, differentiation, and DNA methylation. Cytogenet. Genome Res. *14*, 9–25.

Riley, T., Sontag, E., Chen, P., and Levine, A. (2008). Transcriptional control of human p53-regulated genes. Nat. Rev. Mol. Cell Biol. *9*, 402–412.

Robinson, P.J.J., Fairall, L., Huynh, V.A.T., and Rhodes, D. (2006). EM measurements define the dimensions of the "30-nm" chromatin fiber: evidence for a compact, interdigitated structure. Proc. Natl. Acad. Sci. U. S. A. *103*, 6506–6511.

Rocco, J.W., Leong, C.O., Kuperwasser, N., DeYoung, M.P., and Ellisen, L.W. (2006). p63 mediates survival in squamous cell carcinoma by suppression of p73-dependent apoptosis. Cancer Cell *9*, 45–56.

De Rosa, L., Antonini, D., Ferone, G., Russo, M.T., Yu, P.B., Han, R., and Missero, C. (2009). P63 suppresses non-epidermal lineage markers in a bone morphogenetic protein-dependent manner via repression of Smad7. J. Biol. Chem. *284*, 30574–30582.

Sabari, B.R., Dall'Agnese, A., Boija, A., Klein, I.A., Coffey, E.L., Shrinivas, K., Abraham, B.J., Hannett, N.M., Zamudio, A. V, Manteiga, J.C., et al. (2018). Coactivator condensation at super-enhancers links phase separation and gene control. Science *361*.

Sakata, K., Hoshiyama, Y., Morioka, S., Hashimoto, T., Takeshita, T., and Tamakoshi, A. (2005). Smoking, alcohol drinking and esophageal cancer: findings from the JACC Study. J. Epidemiol. *15 Suppl* 2, S212-9.

Sanchez, R., and Zhou, M.M. (2009). The role of human bromodomains in chromatin biology and gene transcription. Curr. Opin. Drug Discov. Dev. *12*, 659–665.

Santos-Rosa, H., Schneider, R., Bannister, A.J., Sherriff, J., Bernstein, B.E., Emre, N.C.T., Schreiber, S.L., Mellor, J., and Kouzarides, T. (2002). Active genes are tri-methylated at K4 of histone H3. Nature *419*, 407–411.

Sawada, G., Niida, A., Uchi, R., Hirata, H., Shimamura, T., Suzuki, Y., Shiraishi, Y., Chiba, K., Imoto, S., Takahashi, Y., et al. (2016). Genomic Landscape of Esophageal Squamous Cell Carcinoma in a Japanese Population. Gastroenterology *150*, 1171–1182.

Sawyers, C. (2004). Targeted cancer therapy. Nature *432*, 294–297.

Scanlan, M.J., Altorki, N.K., Gure, A.O., Williamson, B., Jungbluth, A., Chen, Y.T., and Old, L.J. (2000). Expression of cancer-testis antigens in lung cancer: Definition of bromodomain testis-specific gene (BRDT) as a new CT gene, CT9. Cancer Lett. *150*, 155–164.

Schmale, H., and Bamberger, C. (1997). A novel protein with strong homology to the tumor suppressor p53. Oncogene *15*, 1363–1367.

Schmitt, A.D., Hu, M., Jung, I., Xu, Z., Qiu, Y., Tan, C.L., Li, Y., Lin, S., Lin, Y., Barr, C.L., et al. (2016). A Compendium of Chromatin Contact Maps Reveals Spatially

Active Regions in the Human Genome. Cell Rep. *17*, 2042–2059.

Schoenfelder, S., Furlan-Magaril, M., Mifsud, B., Tavares-Cadete, F., Sugar, R., Javierre, B.M., Nagano, T., Katsman, Y., Sakthidevi, M., Wingett, S.W., et al. (2015). The pluripotent regulatory circuitry connecting promoters to their long-range interacting elements. Genome Res. *25*, 582–597.

Segura, M.F., Fontanals-Cirera, B., Gaziel-Sovran, A., Guijarro, M. V, Hanniford, D., Zhang, G., González-Gomez, P., Morante, M., Jubierre, L., Zhang, W., et al. (2013). BRD4 sustains melanoma proliferation and represents a new target for epigenetic therapy. Cancer Res. *73*, 6264–6276.

Seitz, H.K., and Stickel, F. (2007). Molecular mechanisms of alcohol-mediated carcinogenesis. Nat. Rev. Cancer *7*, 599–612.

Sen, M., Wang, X., Hamdan, F.H., Rapp, J., Eggert, J., Kosinsky, R.L., Wegwitz, F., Kutschat, A.P., Younesi, F.S., Gaedcke, J., et al. (2019). ARID1A facilitates KRAS signaling-regulated enhancer activity in an AP1-dependent manner in colorectal cancer cells. Clin. Epigenetics *11*, 92.

Servant, N., Varoquaux, N., Lajoie, B.R., Viara, E., Chen, C.J., Vert, J.P., Heard, E., Dekker, J., and Barillot, E. (2015). HiC-Pro: An optimized and flexible pipeline for Hi-C data processing. Genome Biol. *16*.

Seto, E., and Yoshida, M. (2014). Erasers of histone acetylation: The histone deacetylase enzymes. Cold Spring Harb. Perspect. Biol. *6*.

Shah, M.A., Bang, Y.-J., Lordick, F., Alsina, M., Chen, M., Hack, S.P., Bruey, J.M., Smith, D., McCaffery, I., Shames, D.S., et al. (2017). Effect of Fluorouracil, Leucovorin, and Oxaliplatin With or Without Onartuzumab in HER2-Negative, MET-Positive Gastroesophageal Adenocarcinoma: The METGastric Randomized Clinical Trial. JAMA Oncol. *3*, 620–627.

Shang, E., Nickerson, H.D., Wen, D., Wang, X., and Wolgemuth, D.J. (2007). The first bromodomain of Brdt, a testis-specific member of the BET sub-family of double-bromodomain-containing proteins, is essential for male germ cell differentiation. Development *134*, 3507–3515.

Shang, E., Wang, X., Wen, D., Greenberg, D.A., and Wolgemuth, D.J. (2009). Double bromodomain-containing gene Brd2 is essential for embryonic development in Mouse. Dev. Dyn. *238*, 908–917.

Sherr, C.J., and Roberts, J.M. (2004). Living with or without cyclins and cyclin-dependent kinases. Genes Dev. *18*, 2699–2711.

Shi, C., Zhang, H., Wang, P., Wang, K., Xu, D., Wang, H., Yin, L., Zhang, S., and Zhang, Y. (2019). PROTAC induced-BET protein degradation exhibits potent anti-osteosarcoma activity by triggering apoptosis. Cell Death Dis. *10*, 1–11.

Shi, J., Wang, Y., Zeng, L., Wu, Y., Deng, J., Zhang, Q., Lin, Y., Li, J., Kang, T., Tao, M., et al. (2014). Disrupting the Interaction of BRD4 with Diacetylated Twist Suppresses Tumorigenesis in Basal-like Breast Cancer. Cancer Cell *25*, 210–225.

Shi, Y., Lan, F., Matson, C., Mulligan, P., Whetstine, J.R., Cole, P.A., Casero, R.A., and Shi, Y. (2004). Histone demethylation mediated by the nuclear amine oxidase homolog LSD1. Cell *119*, 941–953.

Shilatifard, A. (2012). The COMPASS family of histone H3K4 methylases: Mechanisms of regulation in development and disease pathogenesis. Annu. Rev. Biochem. *81*, 65–95.

Shu, S., Lin, C.Y., He, H.H., Witwicki, R.M., Tabassum, D.P., Roberts, J.M., Janiszewska, M., Huh, S.J., Liang, Y., Ryan, J., et al. (2016). Response and resistance to BET bromodomain inhibitors in triple-negative breast cancer. Nature *529*, 413–417.

Siegel, R.L., Miller, K.D., and Jemal, A. (2019). Cancer statistics, 2019. CA. Cancer J. Clin. *69*, 7–34.

Simonis, M., Klous, P., Splinter, E., Moshkin, Y., Willemsen, R., De Wit, E., Van Steensel, B., and De Laat, W. (2006). Nuclear organization of active and inactive chromatin domains uncovered by chromosome conformation capture-on-chip (4C). Nat. Genet. *38*, 1348–1354.

Simpson, A.J.G., Caballero, O.L., Jungbluth, A., Chen, Y.T., and Old, L.J. (2005). Cancer/testis antigens, gametogenesis and cancer. Nat. Rev. Cancer *5*, 615–625.

Sinha, A., Faller, D. V., and Denis, G. V. (2005). Bromodomain analysis of Brd2-dependent transcriptional activation of cyclin A. Biochem. J. *387*, 257–269.

Smyth, E.C., Lagergren, J., Fitzgerald, R.C., Lordick, F., Shah, M.A., Lagergren, P., and Cunningham, D. (2017). Oesophageal cancer. Nat. Rev. Dis. Prim. *3*, 17048.

Sniezek, J.C., Matheny, K.E., Westfall, M.D., and Pietenpol, J.A. (2004). Dominant negative p63 isoform expression in head and neck squamous cell carcinoma. Laryngoscope *114*, 2063–2072.

Somerville, T.D.D., Xu, Y., Miyabayashi, K., Tiriac, H., Cleary, C.R., Maia-Silva, D., Milazzo, J.P., Tuveson, D.A., and Vakoc, C.R. (2018). TP63-Mediated Enhancer Reprogramming Drives the Squamous Subtype of Pancreatic Ductal Adenocarcinoma. Cell Rep. *25*, 1741-1755.e7.

Song, Y., Li, L., Ou, Y., Gao, Z., Li, E., Li, X., Zhang, W., Wang, J., Xu, L., Zhou, Y., et al. (2014). Identification of genomic alterations in oesophageal squamous cell cancer. Nature *509*, 91–95.

Stadhouders, R., Filion, G.J., and Graf, T. (2019). Transcription factors and 3D genome conformation in cell-fate decisions. Nature *569*, 345–354.

Stahl, M., Stuschke, M., Lehmann, N., Meyer, H.-J., Walz, M.K., Seeber, S., Klump, B., Budach, W., Teichmann, R., Schmitt, M., et al. (2005). Chemoradiation with and without surgery in patients with locally advanced squamous cell carcinoma of the esophagus. J. Clin. Oncol. Off. J. Am. Soc. Clin. Oncol. *23*, 2310–2317.

Stathis, A., and Bertoni, F. (2018). BET proteins as targets for anticancer treatment.

Cancer Discov. *8*, 24–36.

Stevens, H.P., Kelsell, D.P., Bryant, S.P., Bishop, D.T., Spurr, N.K., Weissenbach, J., Marger, D., Marger, R.S., and Leigh, I.M. (1996). Linkage of an American pedigree with palmoplantar keratoderma and malignancy (palmoplantar ectodermal dysplasia type III) to 17q24. Literature survey and proposed updated classification of the keratodermas. Arch. Dermatol. *132*, 640–651.

Subramanian, A., Tamayo, P., Mootha, V.K., Mukherjee, S., Ebert, B.L., Gillette, M.A., Paulovich, A., Pomeroy, S.L., Golub, T.R., Lander, E.S., et al. (2005). Gene set enrichment analysis: A knowledge-based approach for interpreting genome-wide expression profiles. Proc. Natl. Acad. Sci. U. S. A. *102*, 15545–15550.

Suh, E.-K.K., Yang, A., Kettenbach, A., Bamberger, C., Michaelis, A.H., Zhu, Z., Elvin, J.A., Bronson, R.T., Crum, C.P., and McKeon, F. (2006). p63 protects the female germ line during meiotic arrest. Nature *444*, 624–628.

Sun, X., Gao, H., Yang, Y., He, M., Wu, Y., Song, Y., Tong, Y., and Rao, Y. (2019). Protacs: Great opportunities for academia and industry. Signal Transduct. Target. Ther. *4*, 1–33.

Takahashi, K., and Yamanaka, S. (2006). Induction of pluripotent stem cells from mouse embryonic and adult fibroblast cultures by defined factors. Cell *126*, 663–676.

Takeshita, K., Suetake, I., Yamashita, E., Suga, M., Narita, H., Nakagawa, A., and Tajima, S. (2011). Structural insight into maintenance methylation by mouse DNA methyltransferase 1 (Dnmt1). Proc. Natl. Acad. Sci. U. S. A. *108*, 9055–9059.

Tam, V., Patel, N., Turcotte, M., Bossé, Y., Paré, G., and Meyre, D. (2019). Benefits and limitations of genome-wide association studies. Nat. Rev. Genet. *20*, 467–484.

Tanaka, Y., Naruse, I., Hongo, T., Xu, M.J., Nakahata, T., Maekawa, T., and Ishii, S. (2000). Extensive brain hemorrhage and embryonic lethality in a mouse null mutant of CREB-binding protein. Mech. Dev. *95*, 133–145.

Tanner, K.G., Langer, M.R., and Denu, J.M. (2000). Kinetic mechanism of human histone acetyltransferase P/CAF. Biochemistry *39*, 11961–11969.

Taylor, P.R., Li, B., Dawsey, S.M., Li, J.Y., Yang, C.S., Guo, W., and Blot, W.J. (1994). Prevention of esophageal cancer: the nutrition intervention trials in Linxian, China. Linxian Nutrition Intervention Trials Study Group. Cancer Res. *54*, 2029s-2031s.

Tenney, K., and Shilatifard, A. (2005). A COMPASS in the voyage of defining the role of trithorax/MLL-containing complexes: Linking leukemogensis to covalent modifications of chromatin. J. Cell. Biochem. *95*, 429–436.

Tonekaboni, S.A.M., Mazrooei, P., Kofia, V., Haibe-Kains, B., and Lupien, M. (2019). Identifying clusters of cis-regulatory elements underpinning TAD structures and lineage-specific regulatory networks. Genome Res. *29*, 1733–1743.

Toyota, M., and Issa, J.P.J. (2005). Epigenetic changes in solid and hematopoietic tumors. Semin. Oncol. *32*, 521–530.

Tran, G.D., Sun, X.-D., Abnet, C.C., Fan, J.-H., Dawsey, S.M., Dong, Z.-W., Mark, S.D., Qiao, Y.-L., and Taylor, P.R. (2005). Prospective study of risk factors for esophageal and gastric cancers in the Linxian general population trial cohort in China. Int. J. Cancer *113*, 456–463.

Traversari, C., Bruggen, P. van der, Luescher, I.F., Lurquin, C., Chomez, P., Pel, A. Van, Plaen, E. De, Amar-Costesec, A., and Boon, T. (1992). A nonapeptide encoded by human gene MAGE-1 is recognized on HLAA1 by cytolytic t lymphocytes directed against tumor antigen MZ2-E. J. Exp. Med. *176*, 1453–1457.

Trievel, R.C., Rojas, J.R., Sterner, D.E., Venkataramani, R.N., Wang, L., Zhou, J., Allis, C.D., Berger, S.L., and Marmorstein, R. (1999). Crystal structure and mechanism of histone acetylation of the yeast GCN5 transcriptional coactivator. Proc. Natl. Acad. Sci. U. S. A. *96*, 8931–8936.

Trink, B., Okami, K., Wu, L., Sriuranpong, V., Jen, J., and Sidransky, D. (1998). A new human p53 homologue. Nat. Med. *4*, 747–748.

Trivers, K.F., Sabatino, S.A., and Stewart, S.L. (2008). Trends in esophageal cancer incidence by histology, United States, 1998-2003. Int. J. Cancer *123*, 1422–1428.

Tse, C., Sera, T., Wolffe, A.P., and Hansen, J.C. (1998). Disruption of Higher-Order Folding by Core Histone Acetylation Dramatically Enhances Transcription of Nucleosomal Arrays by RNA Polymerase III. Mol. Cell. Biol. *18*, 4629–4638.

Tse, G.M., Tan, P.H., Chaiwun, B., Puttis, T.C., Lui, P.C.W., Tsang, A.K.H., Wong, F.C.L., and Lo, A.W.I. (2006). p63 is useful in the diagnosis of mammary metaplastic carcinomas. Pathology *38*, 16–20.

Uebelacker, M., and Lachenmeier, D.W. (2011). Quantitative determination of acetaldehyde in foods using automated digestion with simulated gastric fluid followed by headspace gas chromatography. J. Autom. Methods Manag. Chem. *2011*, 907317.

Ullrich, A., and Schlessinger, J. (1990). Signal transduction by receptors with tyrosine kinase activity. Cell *61*, 203–212.

Umehara, T., Nakamura, Y., Jang, M.K., Nakano, K., Tanaka, A., Ozato, K., Padmanabhan, B., and Yokoyama, S. (2010). Structural basis for acetylated histone H4 recognition by the human BRD2 bromodomain. J. Biol. Chem. *285*, 7610–7618.

Vaughan, T.L., Davis, S., Kristal, A., and Thomas, D.B. (1995). Obesity, alcohol, and tobacco as risk factors for cancers of the esophagus and gastric cardia: adenocarcinoma versus squamous cell carcinoma. Cancer Epidemiol. Biomarkers Prev. a Publ. Am. Assoc. Cancer Res. Cosponsored by Am. Soc. Prev. Oncol. *4*, 85–92.

Venter, J.C., Adams, M.D., Myers, E.W., Li, P.W., Mural, R.J., Sutton, G.G., Smith, H.O., Yandell, M., Evans, C.A., Holt, R.A., et al. (2001). The Sequence of the Human Genome. Science (80-.). *291*, 1304 LP – 1351.

Vioque, J., Barber, X., Bolumar, F., Porta, M., Santibáñez, M., de la Hera, M.G., and Moreno-Osset, E. (2008). Esophageal cancer risk by type of alcohol drinking and smoking: a case-control study in Spain. BMC Cancer *8*, 221.

Vultos, F., Fernandes, C., Mendes, F., Marques, F., Correia, J.D.G., Santos, I., and Gano, L. (2017). A Multifunctional Radiotheranostic Agent for Dual Targeting of Breast Cancer Cells. ChemMedChem *12*, 1103–1107.

Waddington, C.H. (1942). The epigenotype. Endeavour *1*, 18–20.

Wai, D.C.C., Szyszka, T.N., Campbell, A.E., Kwong, C., Lorna, E.W.W., Silva, A.P.G., Low, J.K.K., Kwan, A.H., Gamsjaeger, R., Chalmers, J.D., et al. (2018). The BRD3 ET domain recognizes a short peptide motif through a mechanism that is conserved across chromatin remodelers and transcriptional regulators. J. Biol. Chem. *293*, 7160–7175.

Walport, L.J., Hopkinson, R.J., Vollmar, M., Madden, S.K., Gileadi, C., Oppermann, U., Schofield, C.J., and Johansson, C. (2014). Human UTY(KDM6C) is a male-specific Nϵ-methyl lysyl demethylase. J. Biol. Chem. *289*, 18302–18313.

Wang, L., and Wolgemuth, D.J. (2016). BET Protein BRDT Complexes with HDAC1, PRMT5, and TRIM28 and Functions in Transcriptional Repression during Spermatogenesis. J. Cell. Biochem. *117*, 1429–1437.

Wang, L.-D., Zhou, F.-Y., Li, X.-M., Sun, L.-D., Song, X., Jin, Y., Li, J.-M., Kong, G.-Q., Qi, H., Cui, J., et al. (2010). Genome-wide association study of esophageal squamous cell carcinoma in Chinese subjects identifies susceptibility loci at PLCE1 and C20orf54. Nat. Genet. *42*, 759–763.

Wang, S., Su, J.H., Beliveau, B.J., Bintu, B., Moffitt, J.R., Wu, C.T., and Zhuang, X. (2016). Spatial organization of chromatin domains and compartments in single chromosomes. Science (80-.). *353*, 598–602.

Watanabe, H., Ma, Q., Peng, S., Adelmant, G., Swain, D., Song, W., Fox, C., Francis, J.M., Pedamallu, C.S., DeLuca, D.S., et al. (2014). SOX2 and p63 colocalize at genetic loci in squamous cell carcinomas. J. Clin. Invest. *124*, 1636–1645.

Wells, A., Kopp, N., Xu, X., O'Brien, D.R., Yang, W., Nehorai, A., Adair-Kirk, T.L., Kopan, R., and Dougherty, J.D. (2015). The anatomical distribution of genetic associations. Nucleic Acids Res. *43*, 10804–10820.

Whyte, W.A., Orlando, D.A., Hnisz, D., Abraham, B.J., Lin, C.Y., Kagey, M.H., Rahl, P.B., Lee, T.I., and Young, R.A. (2013). Master transcription factors and mediator establish super-enhancers at key cell identity genes. Cell *153*, 307–319.

Winter, G.E., Buckley, D.L., Paulk, J., Roberts, J.M., Souza, A., Dhe-Paganon, S., and Bradner, J.E. (2015). DRUG DEVELOPMENT. Phthalimide conjugation as a strategy for in vivo target protein degradation. Science *348*, 1376–1381.

Winter, G.E., Mayer, A., Buckley, D.L., Erb, M.A., Roderick, J.E., Vittori, S., Reyes, J.M., di Iulio, J., Souza, A., Ott, C.J., et al. (2017). BET Bromodomain Proteins

Function as Master Transcription Elongation Factors Independent of CDK9 Recruitment. Mol. Cell *67*, 5-18.e19.

Wolffe, A.P. (2001). Chromatin remodeling: Why it is important in cancer. Oncogene *20*, 2988–2990.

Wu, C.T., and Morris, J.R. (2001). Genes, genetics, and epigenetics: A correspondence. Science (80-.). *293*, 1103–1105.

Wu, C., Hu, Z., He, Z., Jia, W., Wang, F., Zhou, Y., Liu, Z., Zhan, Q., Liu, Y., Yu, D., et al. (2011). Genome-wide association study identifies three new susceptibility loci for esophageal squamous-cell carcinoma in Chinese populations. Nat. Genet. *43*, 679–684.

Wu, C., Kraft, P., Zhai, K., Chang, J., Wang, Z., Li, Y., Hu, Z., He, Z., Jia, W., Abnet, C.C., et al. (2012a). Genome-wide association analyses of esophageal squamous cell carcinoma in Chinese identify multiple susceptibility loci and gene-environment interactions. Nat. Genet. *44*, 1090–1097.

Wu, C., Wang, Z., Song, X., Feng, X.-S., Abnet, C.C., He, J., Hu, N., Zuo, X.-B., Tan, W., Zhan, Q., et al. (2014). Joint analysis of three genome-wide association studies of esophageal squamous cell carcinoma in Chinese populations. Nat. Genet. *46*, 1001–1006.

Wu, M., Liu, A.-M., Kampman, E., Zhang, Z.-F., Van't Veer, P., Wu, D.-L., Wang, P.-H., Yang, J., Qin, Y., Mu, L.-N., et al. (2009). Green tea drinking, high tea temperature and esophageal cancer in high- and low-risk areas of Jiangsu Province, China: a population-based case-control study. Int. J. Cancer *124*, 1907–1913.

Wu, X., Zhang, J., Zhen, R., Lv, J., Zheng, L., Su, X., Zhu, G., Gavine, P.R., Xu, S., Lu, S., et al. (2012b). Trastuzumab anti-tumor efficacy in patient-derived esophageal squamous cell carcinoma xenograft (PDECX) mouse models. J. Transl. Med. *10*, 180.

Xibib, S., Meilan, H., Moller, H., Evans, H.S., Dixin, D., Wenjie, D., and Jianbang, L. (2003). Risk factors for oesophageal cancer in Linzhou, China: a case-control study. Asian Pac. J. Cancer Prev. *4*, 119–124.

Xie, J.J., Jiang, Y.Y., Jiang, Y., Li, C.Q., Lim, M.C., An, O., Mayakonda, A., Ding, L.W., Long, L., Sun, C., et al. (2018). Super-Enhancer-Driven Long Non-Coding RNA LINC01503, Regulated by TP63, Is Over-Expressed and Oncogenic in Squamous Cell Carcinoma. Gastroenterology *154*, 2137-2151.e1.

Yamaji, T., Inoue, M., Sasazuki, S., Iwasaki, M., Kurahashi, N., Shimazu, T., and Tsugane, S. (2008). Fruit and vegetable consumption and squamous cell carcinoma of the esophagus in Japan: the JPHC study. Int. J. Cancer *123*, 1935–1940.

Yan, Y., Barlev, N.A., Haley, R.H., Berger, S.L., and Marmorstein, R. (2000). Crystal structure of yeast Esa1 suggests a unified mechanism for catalysis and substrate binding by histone acetyltransferases. Mol. Cell *6*, 1195–1205.

Yang, C.S. (1980). Research on Esophageal Cancer in China: a Review. Cancer

Res. *40*, 2633 LP – 2644.

Yang, A., and McKeon, F. (2000). p63 and p73: p53 mimics, menaces and more. Nat. Rev. Mol. Cell Biol. *1*, 199–207.

Yang, A., Kaghad, M., Wang, Y., Gillett, E., cell, M.F.-M., and 1998, undefined p63, a p53 homolog at 3q27–29, encodes multiple products with transactivating, death-inducing, and dominant-negative activities. Elsevier.

Yang, A., Schweitzer, R., Sun, D., Kaghad, M., Walker, N., Bronson, R.T., Tabin, C., Sharpe, A., Caput, D., Crum, C., et al. (1999). p63 is essential for regenerative proliferation in limb, craniofacial and epithelial development. Nature *398*, 714–718.

Yang, A., Zhu, Z., Kapranov, P., McKeon, F., Church, G.M., Gingeras, T.R., and Struhl, K. (2006). Relationships between p63 binding, DNA sequence, transcription activity, and biological function in human cells. Mol. Cell *24*, 593–602.

Yang, Z., Yik, J.H.N., Chen, R., He, N., Moon, K.J., Ozato, K., and Zhou, Q. (2005). Recruitment of P-TEFb for stimulation of transcriptional elongation by the bromodomain protein Brd4. Mol. Cell *19*, 535–545.

Ye, J., Coulouris, G., Zaretskaya, I., Cutcutache, I., Rozen, S., and Madden, T.L. (2012). Primer-BLAST: a tool to design target-specific primers for polymerase chain reaction. BMC Bioinformatics *13*, 134.

Yokoyama, A., Lin, M., Naresh, A., Kitabayashi, I., and Cleary, M.L. (2010). A Higher-Order Complex Containing AF4 and ENL Family Proteins with P-TEFb Facilitates Oncogenic and Physiologic MLL-Dependent Transcription. Cancer Cell *17*, 198–212.

Yokoyama, T., Yokoyama, A., Kato, H., Tsujinaka, T., Muto, M., Omori, T., Haneda, T., Kumagai, Y., Igaki, H., Yokoyama, M., et al. (2003). Alcohol flushing, alcohol and aldehyde dehydrogenase genotypes, and risk for esophageal squamous cell carcinoma in Japanese men. Cancer Epidemiol. Biomarkers Prev. a Publ. Am. Assoc. Cancer Res. Cosponsored by Am. Soc. Prev. Oncol. *12*, 1227–1233.

Yuan, J., Jiang, Y.Y., Mayakonda, A., Huang, M., Ding, L.W., Lin, H., Yu, F., Lu, Y., Loh, T.K.S., Chow, M., et al. (2017). Super-enhancers promote transcriptional dysregulation in nasopharyngeal carcinoma. Cancer Res. *77*, 6614–6626.

Yuan, M., Huang, L.L., Chen, J.H., Wu, J., and Xu, Q. (2019). The emerging treatment landscape of targeted therapy in non-small-cell lung cancer. Signal Transduct. Target. Ther. *4*.

Yuan, W., Condorelli, G., Caruso, M., Felsani, A., and Giordano, A. (1996). Human p300 protein is a coactivator for the transcription factor MyoD. J. Biol. Chem. *271*, 9009–9013.

Yun, M., Wu, J., Workman, J.L., and Li, B. (2011). Readers of histone modifications. Cell Res. *21*, 564–578.

Zampieri, M., Ciccarone, F., Palermo, R., Cialfi, S., Passananti, C., Chiaretti, S.,

Nocchia, D., Talora, C., Screpanti, I., and Caiafa, P. (2014). The epigenetic factor BORIS/CTCFL regulates the NOTCH3 gene expression in cancer cells. Biochim. Biophys. Acta - Gene Regul. Mech. *1839*, 813–825.

Zeng, H., Zheng, R., Guo, Y., Zhang, S., Zou, X., Wang, N., Zhang, L., Tang, J., Chen, J., Wei, K., et al. (2015). Cancer survival in China, 2003-2005: a population-based study. Int. J. Cancer *136*, 1921–1930.

Zengerle, M., Chan, K.-H.H., and Ciulli, A. (2015). Selective Small Molecule Induced Degradation of the BET Bromodomain Protein BRD4. ACS Chem. Biol. *10*, 1770–1777.

Zhang, H., Li, G., Zhang, Y., Shi, J., Yan, B., Tang, H., Chen, S., Zhang, J., Wen, P., Wang, Z., et al. (2020a). Targeting BET Proteins With a PROTAC Molecule Elicits Potent Anticancer Activity in HCC Cells. Front. Oncol. *9*, 1471.

Zhang, J., Liu, W., Zou, C., Zhao, Z., Lai, Y., Shi, Z., Xie, X., Huang, G., Wang, Y., Zhang, X., et al. (2020b). Targeting Super-Enhancer–Associated Oncogenes in Osteosarcoma with THZ2, a Covalent CDK7 Inhibitor. Clin. Cancer Res. *26*, 2681–2692.

Zhang, X., Ouyang, S., Kong, X., Liang, Z., Lu, J., Zhu, K., Zhao, D., Zheng, M., Jiang, H., Liu, X., et al. (2014). Catalytic mechanism of histone acetyltransferase p300: From the proton transfer to acetylation reaction. J. Phys. Chem. B *118*, 2009–2019.

Zhang, Y., Liu, T., Meyer, C.A., Eeckhoute, J., Johnson, D.S., Bernstein, B.E., Nussbaum, C., Myers, R.M., Brown, M., Li, W., et al. (2008). Model-based analysis of ChIP-Seq (MACS). Genome Biol. *9*.

Zhao, Y., and Garcia, B.A. (2015). Comprehensive catalog of currently documented histone modifications. Cold Spring Harb. Perspect. Biol. *7*.

Zhao, J., He, Y.-T., Zheng, R.-S., Zhang, S.-W., and Chen, W.-Q. (2012). Analysis of esophageal cancer time trends in China, 1989- 2008. Asian Pac. J. Cancer Prev. *13*, 4613–4617.

Zhao, X.D., Han, X., Chew, J.L., Liu, J., Chiu, K.P., Choo, A., Orlov, Y.L., Sung, W.K., Shahab, A., Kuznetsov, V.A., et al. (2007). Whole-Genome Mapping of Histone H3 Lys4 and 27 Trimethylations Reveals Distinct Genomic Compartments in Human Embryonic Stem Cells. Cell Stem Cell *1*, 286–298.

Zhao, Y., Lu, S., Wu, L., Chai, G., Wang, H., Chen, Y., Sun, J., Yu, Y., Zhou, W., Zheng, Q., et al. (2006a). Acetylation of p53 at Lysine 373/382 by the Histone Deacetylase Inhibitor Depsipeptide Induces Expression of p21Waf1/Cip1. Mol. Cell. Biol. *26*, 2782–2790.

Zhao, Z., Tavoosidana, G., Sjölinder, M., Göndör, A., Mariano, P., Wang, S., Kanduri, C., Lezcano, M., Sandhu, K.S., Singh, U., et al. (2006b). Circular chromosome conformation capture (4C) uncovers extensive networks of epigenetically regulated intra- and interchromosomal interactions. Nat. Genet. *38*, 1341–1347.

Zheng, H., and Xie, W. (2019). The role of 3D genome organization in development and cell differentiation. Nat. Rev. Mol. Cell Biol. *20*, 535–550.

Zhou, Y.B., Gerchman, S.E., Ramakrishnan, V., Travers, A., and Muyldermans, S. (1998). Position and orientation of the globular domain of linker histone H5 on the nucleosome. Nature *395*, 402–405.

www.ingramcontent.com/pod-product-compliance
Lightning Source LLC
LaVergne TN
LVHW041058150826
845673LV00007B/1826
* 9 7 8 3 3 8 4 2 2 2 3 2 9 *